AF443489

Bile Acids in Liver Diseases

Bile Acids in Liver Diseases

EDITED BY

G. Paumgartner and U. Beuers

Department of Medicine II
Klinikum Grosshadern
University of Munich
D-81377 Munich
Germany

*Proceedings of the International Falk Workshop held in Munich, Germany,
January 26–27, 1995*

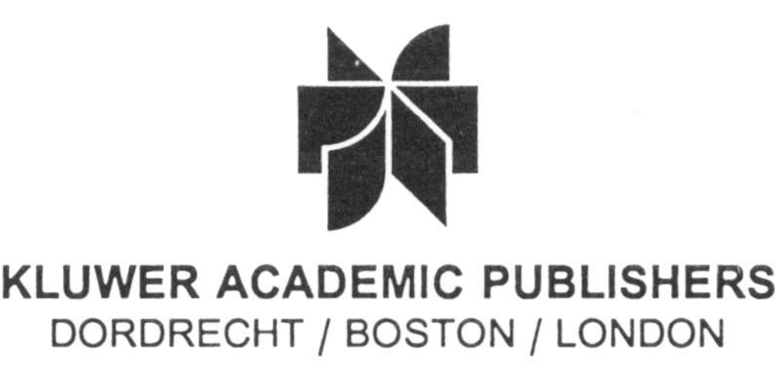

KLUWER ACADEMIC PUBLISHERS
DORDRECHT / BOSTON / LONDON

Distributors

---

for the United States and Canada: Kluwer Academic Publishers, PO Box 358, Accord Station, Hingham, MA 02018–0358, USA
for all other countries: Kluwer Academic Publishers Group, Distribution Center, PO Box 322, 3300 AH Dordrecht. The Netherlands

A catalogue record for this book is available from the British Library

ISBN 0–7923–8891–7

Library of Congress Cataloging in Publication Data

Falk Symposium (1995: Munich, Germany)
    Bile acids in liver diseases: proceedings of the International Falk Workshop held in Munich, Germany, January 26–27, 1995 / edited by G. Paumgartner and U. Beuers.
      p. cm.
    Includes bibliographical references and index.
    ISBN 0–7923–8891–7 (alk. paper)
    1. Liver—Pathophysiology—Congresses. 2. Bile acids—Pathophysiology—Congresses. I. Paumgartner, G. (Gustav) II. Beuers, U. III. Title.
    [DNLM: 1. Bile Acids and Salts—physiology—congresses. 2. Liver Diseases—physiopathology—congresses. 3. Liver Diseases—drug therapy—congresses. 4. Biological Transport—congresses. WI 703 F191bd 1995]
    RC845.F35   1995
    616.3′6207—dc20
    DNLM/DLC
    for Library of Congress   95–24717
                                     CIP

Contents

SECTION III: NEW CONCEPTS OF BILE ACID-INDUCED HEPATOTOXICITY AND BILE SECRETION

SECTION IV: BILE SECRETORY FUNCTION OF LIVER AND BILE DUCT CELLS

SECTION V: URSODEOXYCHOLIC ACID TREATMENT IN CHOLESTATIC LIVER DISEASES

CONTENTS

List of Principal Authors

U. Beuers
Department of Medicine II
Klinikum Grosshadern
University of Munich
Marchioninistr. 15
D-81377 Munich
Germany

J.L. Boyer
Liver Center
Section of Digestive Disease
Yale University School of Medicine
333 Cedar Street
New Haven
CT 06510
USA

J.M. Crawford
Department of Pathology
Brigham and Women's Hospital
75 Francis Street
Boston
MA 02115
USA

C. Gartung
Liver Center
Department of Medicine
Yale University School of Medicine
1080 LMP, PO Box 208019
New Haven
CT 06520-8019
USA

G.J. Gores
Center for Basic Research in Digestive
    Diseases
Mayo Clinic and Mayo Foundation
200 First Street SW
Rochester
MN 55905-0001
USA

S. Güldütuna
Medizinische Klinik II
Abteilung für Gastroenterologie
Zentrum der Inneren Medizin
Klinikum der Universität
D-60590 Frankfurt
Germany

B. Hagenbuch
Division of Clinical Pharmacology and
    Toxicology
Department of Internal Medicine
University Hospital
CH-8091 Zurich
Switzerland

A.F. Hofmann
Division of Gastroenterology
Department of Medicine (0813)
University of California, San Diego
La Jolla
CA 92093-0813
USA

D. Keppler
Deutsches Krebsforschungzentrum
Abteilung Tumorbiochemie
Im Neuenheimer Feld 280
D-69120 Heidelberg
Germany

W. Kramer
Hoechst AG
PGU Metabolism
Postfach 80 03 20
D-65903 Frankfurt am Main
Germany

K.D. Lindor
Mayo Clinic
Mayo Foundation
200 First Street SW
Rochester
MN 55905-0001
USA

R.P.J. Oude Elferink
Department of Gastrointestinal and Liver
  Diseases
AMC, University of Amsterdam
Meibergdreef 9
NL-1105 AZ Amsterdam
The Netherlands

G. Paumgartner
Department of Medicine II
Klinikum Grosshadern
University of Munich
Marchioninistr. 15
D-81377 Munich
Germany

R. Poupon
Unité d'Hepato-Gastroenterologie
Hôpital Saint-Antoine
184 rue du Faubourg Saint-Antoine
F-75571 Paris Cedex 12
France

J. Sjövall
Department of Medical Biochemistry and
  Biophysics
Karolinska Institutet
S-171 77 Stockholm
Sweden

A. Stiehl
Medizinische Universitätsklinik
Bergheimer Str. 58
D-69115 Heidelberg
Germany

M. Strazzabosco
Istituto di Medicina Interna
Universita di Padova
Via Giustiniani 2
I-35100 Padova
Italy

Z.R. Vlahcevic
Division of Gastroenterology
Medical College of Virginia
MCV Station Box 711
Richmond
VA 23298-0711
USA

Preface

During the last decade, bile acid research has attracted increasing attention from both basic scientists and clinical hepatologists. Experimental studies have expanded our knowledge on the role of bile acids in liver disease. Well-designed trials have documented the beneficial effect of bile acid treatment for a number of hepatobiliary diseases.

This book comprises the contributions of an International Falk Workshop devoted to 'Bile Acids in Liver Diseases'. The workshop was held in January 1995 in Munich, preceding the 1995 Annual Meeting of the German Association for the Study of the Liver. In five sessions, leading scientists from eight countries presented an outstanding overview on the current knowledge of bile acid synthesis and metabolism in health and liver disease, bile acid transport and its regulation within the liver, the role of bile acids in bile formation, and new concepts of bile acid-induced hepatotoxicity. Controlled clinical trials demonstrating the beneficial effect of ursodeoxycholic acid in the treatment of a number of cholestatic liver diseases were critically reviewed and the putative mechanism(s) of action of ursodeoxycholic acid were discussed. Thus, the contributions in this book present and discuss the most recent advances in bile acid research and their therapeutic implications. We extend our thanks to the contributors of this volume, to Dr Herbert Falk for his generous support and to Mr Phil Johnstone from Kluwer Academic Publishers for superb cooperation in publishing these proceedings.

Gustav Paumgartner
Ulrich Beuers

Section I
Bile acid synthesis

1
Species differences in bile acid metabolism

A. F. HOFMANN, C. D. SCHTEINGART and L. R. HAGEY

INTRODUCTION

In this chapter we will discuss selected aspects of species differences in bile acid (and bile alcohol) metabolism. Both endogenous and exogenous bile acids will be considered.

Bile acids were among the first biochemicals to be isolated from animal tissues as discrete chemical entities. The isolation of bile acids from animal bile occurred at a time when biochemistry had yet to exist as a formal discipline[1]. Indeed, the concept that natural substances were discrete chemical entities with specific distinctive physicochemical properties was just being advanced by Chevreul, one of the pioneers of lipid biochemistry[2].

The idea that there were species differences in biliary bile acids was advanced very early. 'Chenocholinic acid' was named for the goose, the species from which it was first isolated by Marsson in 1848. Hyodeoxycholic acid (from the pig) in the form of its glycine conjugate, and cholic acid (from the cow) were both described in the previous year, by Strecker. Deoxycholic acid was isolated in 1885 by Latschinoff. Nonetheless, at the turn of the century only cholic acid and deoxycholic acid had been crystallized (for references see refs 3 and 4). In 1907, Hammarsten named the compound that he isolated from polar bear bile 'ursocholsaure'[5]. This compound was clearly distinguishable by taste, melting point, and chemical properties from cholic acid and deoxycholic acid. After the atomic arrangement of the cholane molecule was deduced by Rosenheim and King in the mid-1930s the correct structures of the more common bile acids were assigned[6]. The tradition of isolating species-specific bile acids and bile alcohols from bile has continued up to the present, with new compounds being reported during 1994. As will be developed later in this chapter, it is useful, in our judgement, to divide 'cholanoids' into three major classes: (1) C_{27} bile alcohols; (2) C_{27} bile acids; and (3) C_{24} bile acids. We shall use the term 'cholanoids' as a collective term for these three classes[7]. Haslewood used the term 'bile salts' as a collective term for the conjugates of these three classes, the chemical form in which they are found in bile[8].

The first C_{27} bile alcohol that was identified was scymnol, which was isolated from shark bile in 1898 by Hammarsten[9]. Extensive work on bile alcohols was subsequently pioneered in Japan by Hoshita and Kazuno and their co-workers[10].

Haslewood and his colleagues isolated and established the structure of the more common C_{27} bile acids in 1950[11].

SPECIES DIFFERENCES IN BILE ACID METABOLISM: REASONS FOR STUDY

In vertebrates, marked species differences are considered uncommon for most metabolic pathways, with the exception of xenobiotic metabolism where both type I and type II biotransformations are known to vary widely between species[12,13]. Species differences in xenobiotic detoxification pathways are likely to result from the response to environmental challenges, as occur in plant–animal warfare. One possibility is that the different structures observed in cholanoid evolution took advantage of type I and type II biotransformation enzymes that had already evolved. The most primitive vertebrates form cholanoid structures (hydroxylated sterols) that appear to be the result of such detoxification mechanism (cf. ref. 14). In addition, in more advanced vertebrates, cholanoid biosynthesis results in the formation of an amphipathic molecule with multiple physiological functions, such as induction of bile flow and lipid solubilization. For a cholanoid to be amphipathic, hydroxylation must be restricted to the hydrophilic (α) face of the molecule.

There appear to be several compelling reasons for studying species differences in bile acid metabolism. First, elucidation of physiological and pathophysiological processes requires a thorough knowledge of the participating biochemicals and their physicochemical properties. Second, as already mentioned, bile acids (and probably bile alcohols) are functional, amphipathic molecules, inducing bile flow, and solubilizing lipids in bile and intestinal content in the form of mixed micelles[15,16]. Development of structure–activity relationships requires a thorough knowledge of the chemistry of bile acids including species differences. Third, as advanced by the late Geoffrey A. D. Haslewood of Guys Hospital Medical School, species differences in biliary bile acids can provide information of value in tracing evolutionary relationships between species[8].

Bile acids are also used therapeutically[17], and animal toxicology studies are generally required by regulatory authorities prior to approval for marketing. A knowledge of species differences in bile acid metabolism is required for planning and interpreting the results of toxicological studies. Bile acids are remarkable for showing marked species differences in toxicity. For example, ursodeoxycholic acid (UDCA) is hepatotoxic in rabbits[18], yet is devoid of any toxicity in humans and is in fact used to treat hepatic disease[19,20]. In another remarkable example, cholyltaurine, a common primary bile acid, is hepatotoxic in guinea pigs, yet devoid of toxicity in rats, rabbits and hamsters[21].

BILE ACID METABOLISM

Definition

For cholanoids the term 'metabolism' denotes biosynthesis and biotransformation during enterohepatic cycling. Metabolism also includes active transport by the hepatocyte and enterocyte, and the resultant of intestinal conservation, the circulating (exchangeable) bile acid pool. For primary bile acids (formed in the liver from cholesterol), metabolism includes production (or biosynthesis) rate, as well as the quotient of production rate divided by the pool size, which is the fractional turnover rate. For secondary bile acids (formed in the intestine by bacterial modification of the nuclear substituents of primary bile acids), production rate denotes the amount that is formed from the primary bile acid precursor. The product of production rate and the fraction of that which enters the exchangeable bile acid pool may be defined as 'input' and is analogous to the biosynthesis of primary bile acids. Bile acids are enterohepatic molecules and their tissue distribution is essentially limited to the hepatobiliary system, intestine and plasma. Therefore a description of metabolism includes movements through these 'spaces' which are the result of both transport and flow processes. Finally, for primary bile acids, one is interested in production rate in relation to cholesterol elimination rate, in order to ascertain what fraction of cholesterol is eliminated as bile acids rather than as cholesterol *per se*. Multicompartmental models have been constructed that appear useful to describe quantitatively each of these aspects of cholanoid metabolism[22–24].

Determinants of the chemical composition of the bile acid pool

Because of efficient intestinal conservation, a mass of circulating bile acids moves from biliary tract to intestine during eating, and back into the biliary tract during interprandial periods. This mass can be approximately measured by the technique of isotope dilution[25], as introduced by Lindstedt[26], and is defined as the exchangeable bile acid pool; it is usually just termed the 'pool'.

At least six factors are the major determinants of the chemical composition of the endogenous bile acid pool. These are: (1) the rate of hepatic *de novo* synthesis of individual primary bile acids from cholesterol (formation of the 'mature' molecule); (2) their mode of conjugation; (3) input from the intestine of molecules 'damaged' by bacterial enzymes during enterohepatic cycling; (4) their mode of conjugation; (5) the extent to which such damaged molecules undergo 'repair'; and (6) the efficiency of intestinal conservation of each of the individual bile acids that is secreted into the intestine. Some of these processes may be undetectable by analysis of biliary bile acids. For example, cholanoids can be deconjugated and then reconjugated (or dehydroxylated and rehydroxylated) in such a way that the parent compound is formed once again by hepatic repair.

Bacterial damage can be divided into two major types, in a manner analogous to that proposed by Williams[27] for hepatic biotransformation of drugs. The first type is deconjugation, that is hydrolysis of the bond(s) linking the bile acid to its conjugating compound(s). As discussed later, the common compounds used for bile acid conjugation include taurine, glycine, sulphate and glucuronate.

Uncommon compounds include glucose, *N*-acetylglucosamine, cysteinolic acid, *N*-methyltaurine and dipeptides such as glycyltaurine[15].

The second type of bacterial damage includes 7-dehydroxylation and oxidoreduction of hydroxyl groups. Also included in this type of bacterial biotransformation is desaturation–saturation, a process likely to involve hydrogen atoms adjacent to hydroxyl groups, and which has received relatively little study[28].

The process of 7-dehydroxylation forms new bile acids, which may accumulate in the circulating bile acids; in some species these 7-deoxy bile acids become the predominant bile acid in the bile acid pool. Two examples of such species are the rabbit[29] and the sperm whale[30], in which deoxycholic acid, a secondary bile acid, is the major circulating bile acid. Characterization of faecal bile acids provides information on what kinds of biotransformations can be mediated by the colonic bacteria in a given species. However, faecal bile acid analysis cannot provide information on either the dynamics of bacterial biotransformation or on what intermediates are formed.

Each endogenous bile acid has its individual synthesis rate and its individual efficiency of intestinal conservation. Each individual bile acid has its own pool, and it is the sum of the individual bile acid pools which constitutes the total bile acid pool. Because a substantial fraction of the total bile acid pool is stored in the gallbladder in the fasting-state animal, gallbladder bile is commonly sampled to provide information on the composition of the total bile acid pool.

For exogenous bile acids the same general principles apply. Each administered bile acid will develop its own bile acid pool, the size of which depends on the dose administered, the efficiency of absorption of the administered compound and the efficiency of intestinal conservation of the compound or its hepatic biotransformation products. As with primary bile acids the metabolism of any exogenous bile acid may also involve additional hydroxylation and conjugation, as well as bacterial damage and subsequent hepatic repair.

Sampling the circulating bile acids

Given the dynamic nature of the enterohepatic circulation of bile acids, the investigator wishes to obtain a biological sample that will provide some sort of integrated information. In the fasting state animal the gallbladder is likely to contain a representative sample of the exchangeable bile acid pool, as noted above, since the gallbladder continuously stores a fraction of bile that is secreted during the postprandial period.

In species with gallbladders, bile is readily obtained in an animal that has died spontaneously or has been sacrificed. In humans, bile is obtained by duodenal drainage of bile after the gallbladder has been induced to contract by parenteral administration of cholecystokinin, by gallbladder puncture during surgery, by collection from an external biliary fistula[31], or by percutaneous puncture of the gallbladder[32].

In animals without gallbladders, duct bile may be sampled, but its composition comprises those bile acids just secreted by the liver, a combination of those returning at that moment from the intestine, plus a smaller amount of newly synthesized bile acids.

The second tissue to be sampled is faecal material. Collection of faeces is simple, and faecal analyses provide both qualitative and quantitative information about bile acid metabolism. The chemical composition of faecal bile acids is determined by the pattern of hepatic biosynthesis and subsequent enzymatic action of intestinal bacteria on bile acids.

Biliary cholanoid composition is not identical to the relative rates of input, because individual bile acids or alcohols vary in their efficiency of intestinal conservation (for primary bile acids, input is hepatic biosynthesis; for secondary bile acids, input is absorption of newly formed molecules from the distal intestine). Those bile acids that are more efficiently conserved will develop a larger pool for a given rate of biosynthesis.

To determine cholanoid synthesis rate it must be measured directly. Several methods for quantifying synthesis rate are available.

The first method is measurement of faecal output. Because urinary excretion of bile acids and bile alcohols is believed to be negligible in virtually all vertebrates, faecal excretion of cholanoids is essentially identical to the rate of their hepatic biosynthesis.

The second method for measurement of bile acid synthesis or input is isotope dilution. In this technique the bile acid pool is tagged with a labelled bile acid and either bile[25,26] or plasma (cf refs 33 and 34) is sampled at daily intervals to define the change in specific activity with time.

Bile acid biosynthesis may also be determined by measuring loss of a labelled atom from cholesterol[35,36]. The input of secondary bile acids is usually measured by isotope dilution[24,25,37,38] using samples of bile or plasma.

For a more dynamic description of the metabolism and enterohepatic circulation of bile acids one must sample each 'space' individually. For example, sampling of portal venous blood provides information on species absorbed from the intestine[39]. The composition of systemic venous plasma provides information on the spillover of individual bile acid species into the plasma compartment[40,41]. The composition of small intestinal content at various distances from its origin provides information on absorption and bacterial biotransformation (cf refs 42–44).

Chemical methods for bile acid analysis

The methods used for the chemical identification of bile acids are those of natural product chemistry. For bile acids and bile alcohols, class isolation methods involve liquid/liquid partition, ion-exchange chromatography, gel permeation chromatography and liquid/solid phase adsorption[45]. For individual molecules, separation methods include adsorption chromatography (TLC and column chromatography), and partition chromatography (HPLC and GLC)[46]. Individual structure assignments require NMR and GC/MS (cf refs 47–51). As for any new compound, a synthetic standard is highly desirable. Many of the naturally occurring bile acid epimers have been synthesized during the past decade by Iida and his colleagues[52].

SYSTEMATICS OF CHOLANOIDS IN VERTEBRATES

Biosynthetic pathways

The biosynthesis of C_{24} bile acids is considered to involve two major pathways. The first pathway is the 'neutral' pathway, in which nuclear biotransformations (of cholesterol) are completed before side-chain biotransformations begin; thus, 5β-cholestane-$3\alpha,7\alpha,12$-triol is formed before side-chain hydroxylation or oxidation occurs. The second is the 'acidic pathway' in which side-chain biotransformations are completed before nuclear biotransformations begin (or are limited to 7α-hydroxylation). Here, the side-chain is converted to the structure of isopentanoic acid, while in the nucleus, the 3β-hydroxy-Δ^5 structure of cholesterol remains unchanged. Bile alcohol biosynthesis must be via the neutral pathway, or some variation thereof, since an acidic derivative of the side-chain is never formed. A review of current concepts of the two pathways of C_{24} bile acid biosynthesis has been published[53], and a discussion of their relative importance is included in the contribution of J. Sjövall in Chapter 2 of this volume.

The default cholanoids

Despite there being two pathways of cholanoid biosynthesis the majority of bile acids and bile alcohols that are major biliary species have the following features in the A and B rings: (1) an α-hydroxy group has been added to the C-7 atom; (2) the 3β-hydroxy group has been epimerized to a 3α configuration; (3) the double-bond in the B ring has been eliminated, so that the A and B rings are fully saturated; and (4) the 5-hydrogen atom is in the β configuration with the result that the A/B juncture is *cis*. These processes can be described as 'maturation' of the steroid nucleus.

As mentioned above, we suggest that it is useful to define the simplest structure in each of the three major classes of cholanoids as a 'default' structure. Such default molecules will have a 5β A/B juncture, and 3α- and 7α-hydroxy substituents. For C_{27} bile alcohols the side-chain will be a C_8 branched hydrocarbon chain ending in a terminal C-27 hydroxy group. For C_{27} bile acids the side-chain will be a C_8 branched hydrocarbon chain ending in a terminal C-27 carboxy group. For C_{24} bile acids the side-chain will be a C_5 branched side-chain ending in a terminal C-24 carboxyl group. These structures are summarized in Table 1 and in Fig. 1.

Table 1 The three 'default' cholanoids

Semitrivial name	No. of carbon atoms	Length of side-chain	Terminal functional group	5H configuration	Substituents 3	Substituents 7	Abbreviation
Cholestanetriol	27	C8	OH(C27)	5β	αOH	αOH	chto
Cholestanoic acid	27	C8	COOH(C27)	5β	αOH	αOH	chda
Chenodeoxycholic acid	24	C5	COOH(C24)	5β	αOH	αOH	cdca

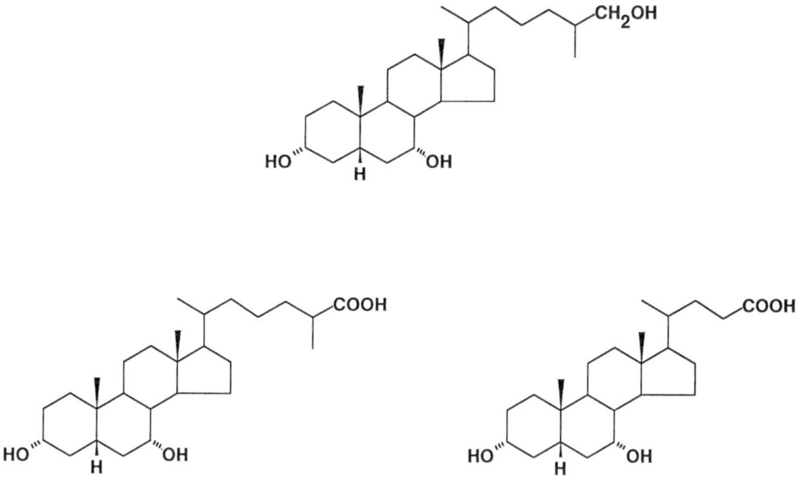

Fig. 1 Chemical structure of the three default cholanoids, the building blocks for most primary bile acids. Top, cholestanetriol; bottom left, cholestanoic acid; bottom right, chenodeoxycholic acid. For more information on structure, see Table 1

Subclasses of the default cholanoids

Unfortunately, subclasses occur in nature which provide exceptions to this attempt at simplification of bile acid systematics. These subclasses have structures differing from those of the default cholanoids in either the steroid nucleus or the side-chain.

The *nuclear subclasses* include those C_{27} alcohols with a 3β-hydroxy group rather than a 3α group. An example is myxinol which occurs in the hagfish. These subclasses also include the 5α (*allo*) bile alcohols and bile acids; these occur in all three default classes[8,54]. Finally, they include substituents other than a 7α-hydroxy group at C-7. For example, in the C_{24} bile acids, $3\alpha,7\beta$-dihydroxy bile acids occur in the Ursidae[55] and the nutria[56], and $3\alpha,7$-oxo bile acids occur in cavimorphs such as the guinea pig[57]. Finally, in boid snakes, biliary bile acids may be lacking *any* substituent at C-7[8,54], suggesting that these bile acids are formed by an 'acidic' pathway in which cholesterol 7α-hydroxylation does not occur. Since all these variations are not exclusive, it is clear that it should be possible to have 16 different subclasses for a given major class. Possible structural variations in molecular structure of the default cholanoids are summarized in Table 2.

The *side-chain subclasses* denote molecules having a double-bond at C22–C23 in the side-chain, as have recently been identified in the mountain paca[58]. In principle, side-chain subclasses may also contain molecules having different chain lengths than C_5 or C_8, or different chain structures (i.e. with alkyl substituents)[59]. For example, C_{26} bile alcohols are common in amphibians. C_{28} bile acids, as also occur in amphibians, may have a precursor other than cholesterol. C_{24} bile alcohols do not occur as major biliary constituents in any species, but are commonly present in trace proportions[60]. The scarcity of C_{24} bile alcohols in bile is a result of the efficient amidation of C_{24} bile acids with taurine or

Table 2 Bile acid biodiversity in vertebrates: classification of variation in molecular structures

		Number of alternatives[a]	*Cumulative number*
I.	Common pathways (major biliary cholanoid in many species)		
	A. Default structures	3	3
	B. Additional hydroxylation	12[b]	36
II.	Uncommon pathways (major biliary cholanoid in 3–12 species)		
	C. A/B ring junction	2	72
	D. 7βOH, 7-oxo, or 7-deoxy	4[c]	216
III.	Rare pathways (major biliary cholanoid in 1–2 species)		
	E. Side chain length	5[b]	864
	F. Side chain saturation	5[b]	4320

[a] Number of alternatives including default structure; the table assumes that all variations can occur independently.
[b] These numbers are crude guesses
[c] $3\alpha,7\beta$-dihydroxy- and 3α-hydroxy, 7-oxo-bile acids have been identified only in C_{24} bile acids

glycine, followed by canalicular secretion. Such biotransformation–excretion precludes reduction of the terminal carboxy group to a terminal hydroxy group, a peroxisomal pathway that is known to occur with long-chain fatty acids during the biosynthesis of complex lipids containing ether bonds such as plasmalogens[61]. As a result of the permutation and combinations of additional hydroxylation, variation in A/B junction, and variation in side-chain length and saturation, there exist several thousand structural possibilities for primary bile acids, as summarized in Table 2.

Subsequent hydroxylation of the cholanoid classes

The default structures may be either secreted as such or may undergo additional hydroxylation on the nucleus, on the side-chain, or on both. Such additional hydroxylation may occur either at any stage of an intermediate during cholanoid biosynthesis or after the mature molecule has been synthesized. This hydroxylation is thought likely to improve the properties of a cholanoid, either by rendering it more soluble, less toxic, or more resistant to bacterial damage (see below).

The rules for subsequent hydroxylation appear to be relatively simple. For C_{27} and C_{24} bile acids there is commonly only one additional hydroxylation on the nucleus or one on the side-chain; rarely is there hydroxylation on *both* the nucleus and the side-chain. Since the default structure has two hydroxy groups, one additional hydroxylation step results in the formation of a trihydroxy bile acid. When hydroxylation occurs on both the nucleus and the side-chain a tetrahydroxy-bile acid is formed; as noted, such bile acids are extremely uncommon as major biliary constituents[54]. Usually hydroxylation is on the polar face (the α face of the molecule) so that the hydrophobic area of the β face is not decreased.

Bile alcohols may undergo one, two, or even three additional hydroxylations before secretion into bile. Since the default structure has three hydroxy groups, biliary bile alcohols are tetrols, pentols or hexols[59].

10

OCCURRENCE OF THE DEFAULT CHOLANOID CLASSES IN VERTEBRATES

C_{27} bile alcohols have long been known to occur in cyclostomes (hagfish, lamprey), cartilaginous fish (sharks, rays), lobe-finned fish (lungfish, coelacanth), and in amphibians (frogs, salamanders)[8]. Recently they have also been identified in bony fish (perciformes)[62]. This laboratory has also reported that C_{27} bile alcohols are the predominant cholanoid in the five ancient mammals (manatee, elephant, rhinoceros, hyrax, and horse)[54]. To date they have not been identified in birds.

C_{27} bile acids have been identified in reptiles and ancient birds. Trace proportions also occur in horses, but C_{27} bile acids have not been reported to occur in other mammals or in fish. C_{24} bile acids occur in modern fish, modern lizards, snakes, modern birds and in mammals[8,54].

The bile of many primitive vertebrates contains both C_{27} bile alcohols and C_{27} bile acids[8]. To explain the persistence of C_{27} bile alcohols despite the ability of the hepatocyte to oxidize the terminal hydroxy group to a carboxyl group, we have proposed the concept of 'organelle competition'; that is, a competition between biotransformation pathways and excretory pathways[62]. In the case of bile alcohols, sulphation, a process mediated by cytosolic enzymes, generates a molecule that is a substrate for canalicular secretion. Thus, sulphation precludes further oxidation of the hydroxy group to a carboxyl group. By the same reasoning, if the terminal hydroxy group of a C_{27} bile alcohol is oxidized to a carboxyl group it can undergo two possible fates. The first is conjugation with taurine and subsequent excretion; the second is transport into peroxisomes, followed by oxidization to a C_{24} bile acid with subsequent conjugation and excretion. This concept is illustrated in Fig. 2. A summary of the occurrence of cholanoid classes in the major orders of vertebrates is given in Table 3.

MOLECULAR SITES OF ADDITIONAL HYDROXYLATION OF DEFAULT CHOLANOIDS AND THEIR OCCURRENCE IN NATURE

Presence of the default cholanoid: no additional hydroxylation

Species that contain only default cholanoids in their bile – that is, with cholanoids whose only sites of hydroxylation are at C-3 and C-7 – are uncommon. Examples for C_{24} bile acids are lemurs, and galliform birds, which may contain only conjugates of CDCA[54].

C_{27} bile alcohols

For C_{27} bile alcohols the C-12 position has long been known as a site for additional (nuclear) hydroxylation[8]. Collaborative work between our laboratory and those of Mosbach and Hoshita established 6-hydroxylation in the manatee[48]. Hydroxylation at C-6 also occurs in the C_{27} bile alcohols of the rock hyrax[54]. Hydroxylation at C-16 occurs in the hagfish (myxinol), and hydroxylation at C-2 occurs in *Arapaima gigas* (a Brazilian fish)[8]. In principle, other sites of hydroxylation on the nucleus could occur.

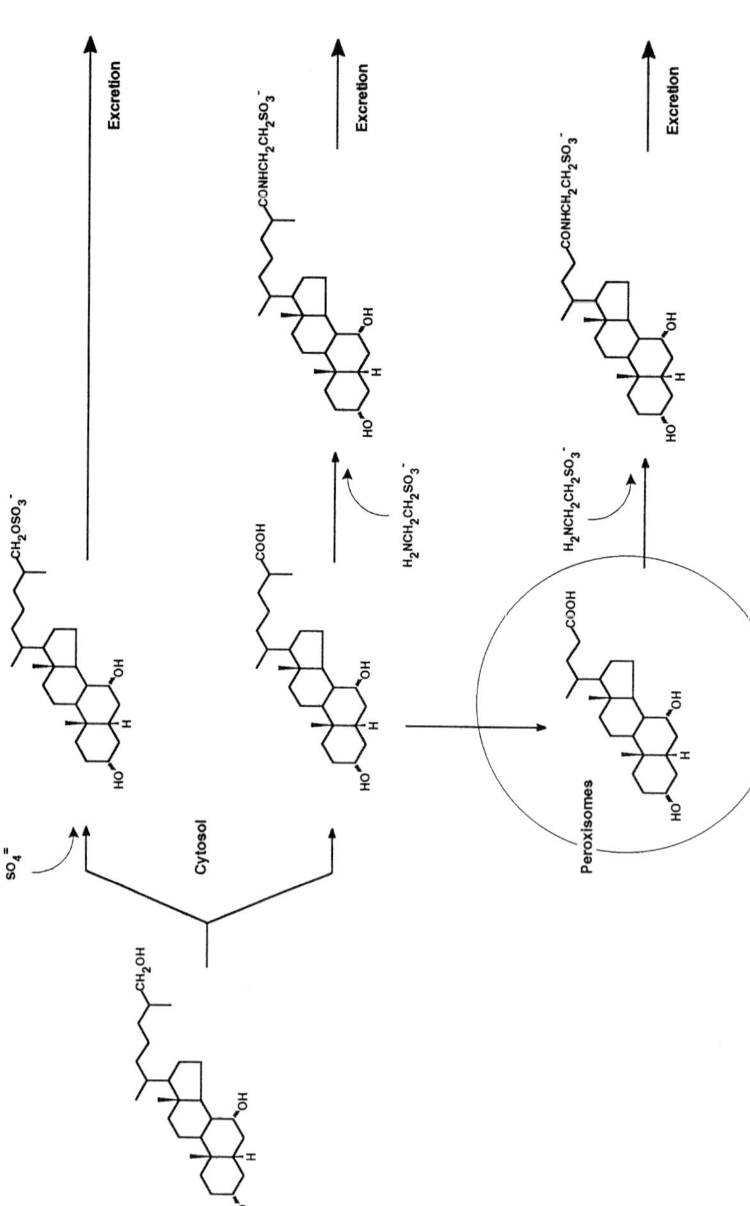

Fig. 2 Concept of organelle competition for cholestanetriol. The compound may be sulphated in the cytosol and then undergo canalicular secretion (excretion). Alternatively, the compound may undergo oxidation in the cytosol to cholestancic acid. This in turn forms a CoA derivative in the cytosol followed by acylation with taurine and subsequent canalicular secretion. Instead of undergoing thio-esterification with CoA, the cholestanoic acid may enter the peroxisomes, undergo side-chain cleavage, and then be conjugated with taurine. It must then be transported out of the peroxisomes to undergo canalicular secretion. Competition for these multiple pathways is likely to be a key determinant of the end-products of cholanoid biosynthesis

Table 3 Predominant bile acid (alcohol) class in major vertebrate classes

		C_{27} alcohols	C_{27} acids	C_{24} acids
I.	Fish			
	Jawless	×		
	Cartilaginous	×		
	Bony fish			
	Lobe-finned	×		
	Ray-finned	×		×
II.	Amphibians			
	Salamanders	×		
	Frogs	×	×	
III.	Reptiles and birds			
	Turtles		×	
	Crocodilians		×	
	Lizards		×	×
	Birds		×	×
	Snakes			×
IV.	Mammals	×	(×)	×

Side-chain hydroxylation (in addition to the default 27-hydroxy group) has been found to occur at one or more carbons on positions 23, 24, 25 and 26[59].

C_{27} bile acids

For C_{27} bile acids, hydroxylation at C-12 has long been established[8], and 16-hydroxylation occurs in the C_{27} bile acids of ancient birds such as vultures and condors[54]. Other sites of additional hydroxylation such as C-1, C-4, or C-6 have not been identified.

Side-chain hydroxylation occurs at C-22 (turtles), C-24 (varanid lizards), C-25 (amphibians) or C-26. Bile acids with two hydroxylation sites on the side-chain have also been reported[59]. Une and Hoshita have recently published a meticulous collation of all known natural C_{27} cholanoids[59].

C_{24} bile acids

For C_{24} bile acids, more information on additional hydroxylation sites is available than for either C_{27} bile alcohols or C_{27} bile acids. Hydroxylation at C-12 and at C-6 has been known for nearly 50 years[3,4]. Hyocholic acid (αOH at C-6) was isolated from porcine bile and its structure assigned by Haslewood and Ziegler (for references see ref. 3). The muricholic acids (βOH at C-6) were isolated from rat bile and the structure of the individual isomers determined by Hsia and other members of the Doisy group[63]. The 7α-hydroxy epimer was termed α-muricholic acid, and the 7β-hydroxy epimer was termed β-muricholic acid. The 7β epimer of hyocholic acid was termed ω-muricholic acid when first isolated, but the bile acid is now called β-hyocholic acid[7]. Hydroxylation at C-16 is now known to be present in many species of birds[54]. Hydroxylation at C-1 (αOH) was identified in the Australian opossum (1α); in fruit doves there is 1β-hydroxylation at C-1[50]. Hydroxylation at C-5 has recently been reported to occur in the pheasant[64]. New sites of 'third' hydroxylation are likely to be discovered. A summary of the sites of

Table 4 Site of the third hydroxy group in C_{24} bile acids

	Nucleus							*Side-chain*	
	1α	*1β*	*5β*	*6α,6β*	*12α*	*15α*	*16α*	*22S*	*23R*
Fish					×			×	
Reptiles									
Lizards					×				
Snakes					×		×		×
Birds		×	×		×		×		×
Mammals									
Marsupial	×				×	×			
Placental				×, ×	×				×

the 'third' hydroxy group is given in Table 4. A list of currently known C_{24} biliary bile acids that occur in bile in concentrations > 2% is given in Table 5.

Side-chain hydroxylation is limited to the $α$ (C-23) or $β$ (C-22) carbon atoms. The 23-hydroxy bile acids are common in snakes, marine mammals and in wading birds[8,54,65], and 22-hydroxy bile acids have been identified in bony fish[66].

CONJUGATION OF BILE ALCOHOLS AND BILE ACIDS

Overview

In virtually all vertebrates, biliary bile acids and bile alcohols are largely present in conjugated form. In contrast to the complexity of bile acid and bile alcohol structure, species differences in conjugation of cholanoids are much fewer. Determinants of the rate of bile acid conjugation include availability of substrate and the substrate specificity of the conjugating enzyme or enzymes. The steady-state pattern of bile acid conjugates observed in bile is determined by the relative rates of conjugation and the relative efficiency of intestinal conservation of each class of conjugates[67].

Conjugation of bile alcohols

Bile alcohols that are major biliary cholanoids are invariably conjugated with one sulphate molecule. The sulphate is believed, on the basis of very limited experimental evidence, to be present on the C-27 hydroxy group[68]. The only known exception occurs in the hagfish, which forms a 3,27 disulphate[8].

Conjugation (*N*-acyl amidation) of bile acids

All C_{27} bile acids that have been characterized have been found to be conjugated with taurine[8,54].

The C_{24} bile acids are also conjugated with taurine in most vertebrates. Rarely, bile acids are conjugated with taurine derivatives. For example, angelfish have *N*-methyltaurine conjugates[54,69], and the red sea bream, a marine teleost, conjugates its bile acids with cysteinolic acid, a hydroxymethyl derivative of taurine, that is present in the algae of its diet[70].

Table 5 Names and structures of C_{24} bile acids (5β-cholanoic acids) in vertebrate bile[a,b]

Semi-trivial name		3	6	7	12	Other	Side-chain	Comment

Position and orientation of substituents:
Nucleus

Semi-trivial name	3	6	7	12	Other	Side-chain	Comment
I. C_{24} Bile acids (5β-cholanoates) with an unsubstituted side-chain							
Chenodeoxycholic acid group[c]							
1. Chenodeoxycholic	α-OH		α-OH				Simplest and common primary BA
2. Ursodeoxycholic	α-OH		β-OH				Primary BA in bear and nutria; 'BP' in other species
3. 7-Oxolithocholic	α-OH		=O				Primary BA in koala and guinea pig
4. Lithocholic	α-OH						B7-DP of 1 and 2
Cholic acid group[c]							
5. Cholic	α-OH		α-OH	α-OH			Common primary BA
6. 7-Epicholic	α-OH		β-OH	α-OH			Can be primary BA in human
7. 7-Oxodeoxycholic	α-OH		=O	α-OH			Can be primary BA in human
8. Deoxycholic	α-OH			α-OH			B7-DP of 5
Hyocholic group							
9. α-Hyocholic	α-OH	α-OH	α-OH				Primary BA in pigs
10. β-Hyocholic	α-OH	α-OH	β-OH				'BP' in rat; originally named ω-muricholic
11. Hyodeoxycholic	α-OH	α-OH					B-7DP of 9; HHP of 3
Muricholic group							
12. α-Muricholic	α-OH	β-OH	α-OH				Primary BA in rodent
13. β-Muricholic	α-OH	β-OH	β-OH				Primary BA in rodent
14. Murideoxycholic	α-OH	β-OH					HHP of 3
Other trihydroxy bile acids[d]							
15. 16α-Hydroxy-CDC	α-OH		α-OH		16α-OH		Primary BA in many birds
16. 16α-hydroxy-DC	α-OH			α-OH	16α-OH		Primary (?) BA in snake
17. 1β-hydroxy-CDC	α-OH		α-OH		1β-OH		Primary BA in pheasant and pigeon
18. 1α-hydroxy-CDC	α-OH		α-OH		1α–OH		Primary BA in Australian marsupials

Table 5 *Continued*

Semi-trivial name	Position and orientation of substituents: Nucleus				Other	Side-chain	Comment
	3	6	7	12			
19. 5β-hydroxy-CDC	α-OH		α-OH		5β-OH		Primary BA in pheasant
20. 15α-hydroxy-CDC	α-OH		α-OH		15α-OH		Primary BA in marsupials
21. 1β-hydroxy-DC	α-OH			α-OH	1β-OH		HHP of 8 in sheep

II. C$_{24}$ bile acids (5β-cholanoates)
with a hydroxy group in the side-chain
23R-Hydroxy-cholic acid group

Semi-trivial name	3	6	7	12	Other	Side-chain	Comment
22. 23R-Hydroxy-C	α-OH		α-OH	α-OH		-23(R)	Primary BA in marine mammals and snakes
23. 23R-Hydroxy-DC	α-OH			α-OH		-23(R)	B7-DP of 22

Other bile acids

Semi-trivial name	3	6	7	12	Other	Side-chain	Comment
24. 23R-Hydroxy-CDCA[d]	α-OH		α-OH			-23(R)	Primary BA in marine mammals and wading birds
25. 22S-Hydroxy-CDCA	α-OH		α-OH			-22(S)	Primary BA in bony fish

III. C$_{24}$ bile acids (5β cholenoates)
with a double bond in the side-chain

Semi-trivial name	3	6	7	12	Other	Side-chain	Comment
26. 7-oxo-litho-Δ^{22}-cholenoate	α-OH			oxo		Δ^{22}	Primary BA in mountain paca
27. Δ^{22}-β-muricholic	α-OH	β-OH	β-OH			Δ^{22}	Primary BA in rats

[a] Abbreviations: C, cholic (acid); CDC, chenodeoxycholic (acid); DC, deoxycholic (acid); BA, bile acid; BP, bacterial product; B7-DP, bacterial 7-dehydroxylation product; HHP, hepatic hydroxylation product. The term 'BP' means that bacteria may form the index compound or generate a precursor that is further metabolized to the index compound by hepatic enzymes.
[b] Nomenclature follows recommendations of a recent consensus statement[7].
[c] 5α (allo) isomers of these bile acids have been identified in some species.
[d] Whether B7-DP of these BA is formed *in vivo* is not known.

Notable exceptions to amidation exclusively with taurine are mammals, in whom glycine conjugates can predominate. Glycine conjugation also occurs in some fruit doves and pigeons[50].

Sulphation of bile acids

Bile acid sulphation does not occur to any appreciable extent in the biliary bile acids of most healthy vertebrates. In humans the secondary bile acid lithocholic acid (formed in the colon by bacterial 7-dehydroxylation of chenodeoxycholic acid) not only undergoes amidation with glycine or taurine on its carboxy group, but also undergoes sulphation at the 3-hydroxy group[71].

In cholestatic liver disease, increased sulphation of primary bile acids occurs in association with increased urinary excretion[72].

Bile acid glucuronidation

Bile alcohol glucuronides are not major biliary constituents in healthy animals. Studies using dihydroxy-bile acids with a modified side-chain, for example C_{23}-nor bile acids or C_{24} α-methyl bile acids, have shown that conjugation with glucuronide occurs when such bile acids are poor substrates for CoA ligase. The lipophilic unconjugated bile acid partitions into the smooth endoplasmic reticulum where it undergoes glucuronidation (with or without additional hydroxylation). Glucuronidation can occur on either the nuclear hydroxy groups (ether glucuronide) or the carboxy group (ester glucuronide)[73].

In humans, hyodeoxycholic acid undergoes efficient (ethereal) glucuronidation at the 6 position[74]; such 6-glucuronidation of this bile acid does not appear to occur in other species. Glucuronides are never major biliary cholanoids because they do not undergo enterohepatic cycling.

The rare inborn error of bile acid biosynthesis, cerebrotendinous xanthomatosis, is caused by absence of the 3,7,12-cholestanetriol 27-hydroxylase, a mitochondrial P450 enzyme[75]. In this disease, large quantities of abnormal bile alcohols are formed with hydroxy groups at C-25 and C-26. These are glucuronidated and eliminated in both urine and bile[76].

Other modes of bile acid conjugation

UDCA has been reported to be conjugated in humans with N-acetylglucosamine[77]. Conjugation with glucose has also been reported[78]. Since these conjugating groups are uncharged, and since efficient biliary secretion requires an anionic charge on the molecule[79], such conjugation is likely to be on a nuclear hydroxy group rather than on the carboxyl group of the side-chain.

Modes of bile acid conjugation are summarized in Table 6.

DAMAGE IN THE ENTERAL LOOP OF THE ENTEROHEPATIC CIRCULATION

Overview

Bile acids are secreted continuously into the small intestine in all animals. A variable fraction of bile that is secreted by the liver is stored in the gallbladder

Table 6   Observed types of bile acid conjugation

	Occurrence
I. Bile acids	
A. Linked to carboxyl group (side-chain)	
1. Taurine	Most vertebrates
2. N-methyltaurine	Angelfish
3. Cysteinolic acid	Fish ingesting algae rich in cysteinolic acid
4. Glycine	Rodents, primates, artiodactylids; pigeons
5. Glucuronate	Nor-dihydroxy bile acids
6. 2-Fluoro-β-alanine	Animals receiving 5-fluorouracil
7. β-Alanine	Taurine-deficient animals
8. Glycyltaurine	Lagomorphs
B. Linked to nuclear hydroxyl group	
1. Sulphate (C-3)	Nor-dihydroxy bile acids
2. Sulphate (C-7)	CDCA in hamsters with cholestasis
3. Glucuronate (C-3)	Nor-dihydroxy bile acids (humans)
4. Glucuronate (C-6)	Hyodeoxycholic acid (humans)
5. Glucose	UDCA (hepatic microsomes)
6. N-acetylglucosamine (C-7)	UDCA (humans)
C. Linked to both carboxyl and nuclear hydroxyl groups	
1. Sulpho (C-3)-amidates (C-24)	LCA in humans; CDCA (cholestasis)
2. Sulpho (C-7)-amidates (C-24)	CDCA (cholestasis)
3. Disulphates or sulphate-glucuronide amidates (C-3 and C-7)	Humans (cholestasis)
II. Bile alcohols	
A. Linked to side-chain hydroxyl group(s)	
1. Sulphate (C-27)	Most vertebrates
2. Glucuronate (not at C-27)	Humans (cerebrotendinous xanthomatosis)
B. Linked to both side-chain and nuclear hydroxyl group(s)	
1. Disulphate (C-3 and C-27)	Myxinol (hagfish)

Several other amino acids have been claimed to be present in biliary bile acids. These include ciliatine (amino-ethane-phosphonic acid), ornithine, and arginine[36]. However, there has been no confirmation of these reports.

(in those species having gallbladders), and the remainder enters the small intestine when the sphincter of Oddi relaxes (in humans, this fraction is about 1/2)[80]. During meals, synchronous gallbladder contraction and relaxation of the sphincter of Oddi evokes the discharge of stored bile acids into the intestine.

Bile acids undergo metabolism by intestinal bacteria. The term 'damage' appears justifiable, as the biotransformation products are unlikely to function as well in lipid transport as their conjugated precursor. Here we will consider three types of damage: (1) deconjugation; (2) 7-dehydroxylation; and (3) oxidoreduction of nuclear hydroxy groups.

Deconjugation

The term 'deconjugation' was originally used to denote hydrolysis of the amide bond between the carboxyl group of the bile acid and the amino acid group of taurine or glycine. Since bile acids may be conjugated with sulphate, glucuronide (or glucose or N-acetylglucosamine), it seems preferable to denote cleavage of the amide bond as 'deamidation'. It could also be termed deacylation when referring to the amino acid moiety.

The colonization of the small intestine by bacteria varies greatly between species. A large variety of bacteria are capable of deamidating C_{24} bile acids, generating the unconjugated bile acid (and glycine or taurine)[81].

In humans, faecal bile acids are present predominantly in unconjugated form[82]. The state of bile acid conjugation in the faeces has been examined in relatively few species to date. The published analyses suggest that, in most species, faecal bile acids are also predominantly in unconjugated form[83]. The unconjugated bile acids that are formed are absorbed to some extent from the small or large intestine, returned to the liver and reamidated, and secreted in bile. The extent to which bile acids are deconjugated and reconjugated during enterohepatic cycling has been measured in only a few species. In the rat, deconjugation and reconjugation have been found to be extensive[84]. In humans the rate of deamidation of glycine amidates is about 100%/day with about 70% of the steroid moiety being conserved and undergoing reconjugation[85]. There are considerable differences between individuals. Taurine amidates undergo less deamidation than glycine amidates during enterohepatic cycling[86]. Bile acids that are conjugated with the N-methyl derivatives of glycine or taurine do not undergo deamidation[87–89].

In humans the sulphate group of sulpholithocholyl amidates is also hydrolysed by bacterial enzymes[90]. Bacterial sulphatases for bile acid sulphates have been characterized in some detail[91]. Presumably the trace amounts of other conjugates (glucuronide, glucose or N-acetylglucosamine) that are excreted in bile also undergo deconjugation by bacterial enzymes.

Dehydroxylation

The one type of bacterial 'damage' that may have a profound influence on biliary bile acid composition is 7-dehydroxylation. This process is mediated by a relatively small number of strictly anaerobic bacteria[92] and is a multiple enzyme process coded by an operon that has been cloned[93]. The process begins with formation of a coenzyme A ester and proceeds through a 3-oxo-Δ^4,Δ^6 intermediate, generating, as final product, a 7-deoxy bile acid[94]. The subsequent processing of the 7-deoxy compound is discussed below.

The process of 7-dehydroxylation occurs only in animals with a caecum, a specialized region of the large intestine in which transit is slow and a strictly anaerobic flora is present. A caecum is present in all herbivorous and omnivorous animals, and in some carnivores. Only unconjugated bile acids undergo 7-dehydroxylation; that is, dehydroxylation of the conjugated moiety occurs far more slowly than deconjugation of the unconjugated moiety. A possible explanation is that the initial step in 7-dehydroxylation is formation of the CoA derivative; such CoA formation does not occur with strong acids such as bile acid amidates or α-hydroxy bile acids. Bile acid sulphonates, in which a sulphonic acid replaces the carboxyl group of the bile acid, also do not undergo 7-dehydroxylation[95].

The extent to which various cholanoids undergo 7-dehydroxylation has not been studied in detail. Bile alcohols are considered to undergo little 7-dehydroxylation. *In vitro* their presence in the reaction medium inhibits 7-dehydroxylation of C_{24} bile acids[96], and 7-deoxy bile alcohols have not been identified in either bile or faeces. Both C_{27} and C_{24} bile acids undergo 7-dehydroxylation.

The A/B ring junction does not appear to influence 7-dehydroxylation, in that *allo* bile acids (such as allocholic acid) readily undergo 7-dehydroxylation[97]. In the guinea pig and koala, biliary bile acids contain $3\alpha,7$-oxo-cholanoic acid, and 7-dehydroxylation occurs nonetheless. Such animals are herbivores with a large caecum, and there is likely to be considerable oxidoreduction at the 7-position permitting the unsaturated intermediate to occur. Bears do not dehydroxylate the 7β-hydroxyl group of ursodeoxycholic acid, as they lack a caecum[55].

Most, but not all, trihydroxy bile acids undergo 7-dehydroxylation. Cholic, 7-epicholic[98] and α-hyocholic[99], readily undergo 7-dehydroxylation. Probably β-hyocholic acid (ω-muricholic acid), α-muricholic acid and β-muricholic acid are relatively resistant to 7-dehydroxylation (cf. refs 100 and 101). Whether bile acids with a 1-hydroxy group (either α or β) undergo 7-dehydroxylation has not been investigated. It is also not known whether C_{24} or C_{27} bile acids with hydroxy groups in the side-chain undergo 7-dehydroxylation. To date the 7-deoxy derivatives of these bile acids have not been identified in either faeces or bile.

Oxidoreduction during enterohepatic cycling

Faecal bile acids contain a wide spectrum of hydroxy-oxo bile acids that are not present in biliary bile acids[82]. This finding indicates that bacterial enzymes mediate the oxidation (dehydrogenation) of nuclear hydroxyl groups to form an oxo group, followed by reduction to either the α or β epimer, these processes being catalysed by bacterial enzymers[102–104]. Dehydrogenation may be mediated by aerobic bacteria and may occur in the small intestine. Based on *in vitro* studies, oxidoreduction can occur without prior deamidation[92].

REPAIR IN THE HEPATIC COMPARTMENT OF THE ENTEROHEPATIC CIRCULATION

Overview

The processes of damage – deconjugation, 7-dehydroxylation and oxidoreduction – are reversed by repair enzymes in the hepatocyte. There is no evidence for repair processes occurring in the enterocyte during transcellular transport.

Reconjugation

Unconjugated bile acids are reamidated during transport through the hepatocyte. The mode of amidation (taurine versus glycine) is approximately similar to that used for conjugation of newly synthesized bile acids. The amino acid transferase prefers to conjugate with taurine, and in humans and rats the extent of conjugation with taurine is directly proportional to hepatocyte taurine concentration[105]. In the majority of adult humans the flux of unconjugated bile acids that undergo reamidation exceeds the flux of newly synthesized bile acids. The same is likely to be true for animals such as the rat in which there is extensive deconjugation of bile acids in the small intestine.

In humans, lithocholic acid is not only amidated, but is also sulphated (at the 3-hydroxy group) to form sulpholithocholyl amidates, as noted above[71].

Rehydroxylation

The 7-deoxy bile acids that return to the liver undergo rehydroxylation to a varying extent that is species-dependent. Rehydroxylation may be at C-7 or at another carbon atom. If rehydroxylation occurs at C-7 the parent compound is formed once again. If rehydroxylation occurs at another site a new bile acid is formed.

Lithocholic acid undergoes efficient 7-rehydroxylation in the guinea pig[21] and hamster[106], but in the rat it undergoes limited 6-hydroxylation[106]. In the rabbit[18] and rhesus monkey[107], lithocholic acid is not rehydroxylated and is merely amidated.

Lithocholic acid is a known hepatotoxic bile acid when administered chronically to animals (reviewed in ref. 18). Despite chenodeoxycholic acid being a very common default cholanoid, and despite its being efficiently converted to lithocholic acid in every species that possesses a caecum, lithocholic acid has never been reported to be present in biliary bile acids in a proportion exceeding 5%, attesting to its efficient detoxification in all vertebrates in which it is formed (for a thorough review of older studies on LCA metabolism and toxicity, see refs 108 and 109).

The hepatic repair of deoxycholic acid is also highly species specific. In the rabbit, deoxycholic acid is not rehydroxylated and it is the dominant biliary bile acid[29]. In humans, deoxycholic acid is also not rehydroxylated[110], and its proportion often exceeds that of cholic acid, its parent compound in older adults[37,111]. In rats there is partial rehydroxylation at C-7[112].

In snakes, $3\alpha,12\alpha,16\alpha$-trihydroxy-cholanoic acid has long been thought to be produced by 16α-hydroxylation of deoxycholic acid[113] which, in turn, had been formed by 7-dehydroxylation of cholic acid. We have reported that some species of boids have no cholic acid in bile[54], raising the possibility that 7-deoxy bile acids are formed in the hepatocyte in these snakes, making the $3\alpha,12\alpha,16\alpha$-trihydroxy bile acid a primary bile acid.

The site of 7-rehydroxylation is presumably microsomal[114]. Since amidation is likely to precede 7-rehydroxylation there must be transport systems that carry the amidates into the luminal side of the endoplasmic reticulum. One of these may be the bile acid transporter described by Levy and his colleagues[115]. The microsomal hydroxylase responsible for 7-rehydroxylation of deoxycholic acid has not been cloned.

Reduction and epimerization

A spectrum of 3α-hydroxy, 3-oxo, 3β-hydroxy and 7β-hydroxy epimers are returned to the hepatocyte in portal blood. The hepatic repair of these 'damaged' bile acids is also highly species-specific.

Based on very limited studies, 3-oxo bile acids are likely to be reduced to the naturally occurring 3α-hydroxy derivative[116]. This process is mediated by the major bile acid binding protein in the cytosol which, at least in some species, has oxidoreductase activity[117]. The guinea pig is an exception. If cholic acid is fed chronically to the guinea pig, the cholic acid is converted to deoxycholic acid which, in turn, accumulates in the circulating bile acids. A fraction of the deoxycholic acid is metabolized to its 3-oxo derivative during hepatocyte transport, and this is secreted into bile[21,118].

The 3β isomers of natural bile acids ('iso' bile acids) are epimerized to the naturally occurring 3α epimers during hepatocyte transport in rats[119,120]. The 7-oxo derivatives of CDCA and cholic acid are reduced stereospecifically, but the direction is species-specific. In dogs[121] and humans[122], 7-oxo bile acids are reduced mostly to the 7α-hydroxy derivative; in rats the reduction is mostly to the 7β-hydroxy derivative[123].

METABOLISM OF EXOGENOUS CHOLANOIDS

Overview

The principles described above can be applied to exogenous cholanoids. Because C_{27} bile alcohols and C_{27} bile acids have never been available in bulk quantities, there are virtually no studies in which these have been fed chronically to animals including humans.

Those bile acids that have been fed chronically to animals including humans are the common, natural bile acids. Although bile acids have generally been administered in unconjugated form, amidates have been administered chronically in a few studies[124–129].

When unconjugated bile acids are administered orally, they are largely absorbed passively from the small intestine, and are not metabolized during passage through the enterocyte and transport to the liver. At the liver they are extracted efficiently from hepatic sinusoidal blood. In contrast to endogenous bile acids, which are always present during their biosynthesis as CoA (thio)esters, exogenous bile acids enter the hepatocyte as an underivatized acid. Whether they form a CoA derivative, and whether the CoA derivative can be acylated with glycine or taurine, is a key determinant of their ultimate metabolism by the hepatocyte[130].

In general, if the exogenous bile acid is efficiently amidated it will be excreted into bile and join the circulating pool of amidates. The degree of enrichment of the bile acid pool by an endogenous bile acid depends on multiple factors including: (a) the input rate of exogenous bile acid compared to that of endogenous bile acid biosynthesis; (b) the efficiency of conservation of the exogenous amidate compared to that of the endogenous amidates; (c) whether the exogenous amidate suppresses the biosynthesis of the endogenous bile acids and/or competes for intestinal conservation of their corresponding amidates; and (d) to what extent the 7-deoxy derivative of the exogenous bile acid accumulates in bile[131].

If, however, the exogenous bile acid does not readily form a CoA derivative, or if its CoA derivative cannot be acylated with glycine or taurine, then its metabolism will differ strikingly from that of endogenous bile acids. Trihydroxy bile acids, such as C_{23} nor-cholic[132] or the 7β-hydroxy and 12β-hydroxy epimer of cholic acid[133], are secreted into bile in unconjugated form. Dihydroxy bile acids are more lipophilic. As a result, unconjugated dihydroxy bile acids are partitioned into the endoplasmic reticulum, where they undergo hydroxylation as well as glucuronidation, followed by secretion into bile[112]. Even if glucuronidation is incomplete, an unconjugated, dihydroxy compound may be directly secreted into bile. Such unconjugated dihydroxy bile acids remain lipophilic, and as a result they are reabsorbed passively from the biliary tract, return to the sinusoids by the periductular capillary plexus, and are once again transported through the hepatocyte and into canalicular bile[130]. Such a cholehepatic circulation will continue until the compound is glucuronidated.

When glucuronidation occurs, the compound is secreted into bile, passes down the biliary tract without being reabsorbed, and enters the small intestine. As noted above, one remarkable exception to these rules is hyodeoxycholic acid, a dihydroxy bile acid, which in humans (but not other animals), is efficiently glucuronidated at the 6-position[74]. As a result, hyodeoxycholic acid does not accumulate in the circulating bile acids when administered chronically to humans[134].

STRUCTURE–FUNCTION RELATIONSHIPS

Overview

We are quite ignorant about structure–function relationships in the evolution of cholanoids. Is a bile alcohol sulphate more suitable for an elephant than cholyltaurine? Is a C_{27} bile acid more suitable for the crocodilians than a C_{24} bile acid? Because the physical properties of the C_{27} cholanoids have never been characterized, we cannot begin to answer these questions.

Consequences of additional hydroxylation of the default cholanoids

In most vertebrates the default cholanoids undergo one or more hydroxylations during biosynthesis. The frequency with which such additional hydroxylation occurs suggests that there is some biological utility to additional hydroxylation of the default cholanoid structure. Hydroxylation is usually on the polar (α) face of the molecule, so that the hydrophobic area of the β face of the molecule is not appreciably diminished. As a result the critical micellar concentration (CMC, a measure of detergency) of trihydroxy bile acids remains essentially unchanged, since the CMC is inversely proportional to the area of the β face of the molecule[135]. Experimental evidence suggests that 5β bile acids are much more soluble at low temperatures than their corresponding 5α derivatives[136]. Such properties might be useful to poikilothermic fish that live in water at subfreezing temperatures.

The effect of adding a 'third' nuclear hydroxy group to chenodeoxycholic acid is to make the molecule slightly more hydrophilic which, in turn, influences its passive membrane permeability[137–139]. If conjugation is incomplete the presence of a third hydroxy group will inhibit cholehepatic shunting[130]. In the small intestine, if deconjugation occurs, the presence of a third hydroxy group decreases the rate of passive absorption[137,138], and thus acts to maintain the intraluminal concentration of bile acids. An additional consequence of adding a third hydroxyl group in the nucleus is to prevent the formation of lithocholic acid; that is, instead of a 3α-hydroxy bile acid being formed, a 3α,X-dihydroxy bile acid is formed, where X is the additional hydroxy group. In general, one would expect 3α,X-dihydroxy bile acids to be less toxic than lithocholic acid.

The addition of an α-carbon (C-23) hydroxy group to the side-chain decreases the rate of deconjugation[140]. In addition it may well decrease the rate of 7-dehydroxylation, since it should be more difficult to form a CoA ester derivative of an α-hydroxy bile acid, because it is a stronger acid than a bile acid with an unsubstituted side-chain.

Consequences of conjugation of cholanoids

Amidation with glycine or taurine has the effect of increasing the bile acid solubility at the slightly acidic pH of the proximal small intestine[141]. Amidation also prevents passive absorption of the bile acid from the biliary tract and small intestine and inhibits its precipitation as an insoluble Ca^{2+} salt. This is because the Ca^{2+} salts of taurine amidates are fully water-soluble, and the Ca^{2+} salts of glycine-conjugated bile acids do not precipitate from solution, even if supersaturation is present[141]. It is noteworthy that amidates of bile acids with most amino acids other than glycine or taurine are rapidly hydrolysed by pancreatic carboxypeptidases[142].

Conjugation of cholanoids with sulphate or glucuronate is likely to increase aqueous solubility and abolish uptake by the bile acid transport system present in the terminal ileum, thus inhibiting enterohepatic cycling. As a result these modes of conjugation serve to eliminate cholanoids from the circulating bile acid pool.

EPILOGUE

This subject of species differences in bile acid biosynthesis and the metabolism of exogenous bile acids is a very large one. The first requirement for gaining a valid perspective of species differences in bile acid metabolism is to characterize in detail the biliary and faecal bile acids of representative vertebrates from the major vertebrate classes. We and others are continuing this classical approach, which appears to be one of the last frontiers of physiological biochemistry. The search is exciting, and continues to yield new molecules. It is hoped that the search will give rise to unifying principles of evolution, and that such principles will give rise in turn to new understandings of bile acid structure–activity relationships. Finally, if we are really fortunate we may be able to find new uses of bile acids in the therapy of hepatobiliary and digestive disease.

Acknowledgements

This work was supported in part by NIH Grant DK 21506 and grants-in-aid from the Falk Foundation e. V., Freiburg, Germany, and Ciba Geigy, Inc. L. R. Hagey was the recipient of the Frank M. Chapman Award from the American Museum of Natural History in 1992.

References

1. Fruton JS. The emergence of biochemistry. Science. 1976;192:327–34.
2. Costa AB. Michel Eugene Chevreul: Pioneer of Organic Chemistry. Madison: The Department of History, University of Wisconsin; 1962.
3. Matschiner JT. Naturally ocurring bile acids and alcohols and their origins. In: Nair PP, Kritchevsky D, editors. The bile acids, chemistry, physiology and Metabolism, Vol. 1. New York: Plenum Press; 1971:11–46.
4. Sobotka H. Physiological chemistry of bile. Baltimore: Williams & Wilkins; 1937.
5. Hammarsten O. Untersuchungen ueber die Gallen einiger Polartiere. III. Mitteilung. Hoppe-Seylers Z Physiol Chem. 1909;61:454–93.
6. Rosenheim O, King H. The ring system of sterols and bile acids. Nature. 1932;130:315.
7. Hofmann AF, Sjövall J, Kurz G et al. A proposed nomenclature for bile acids. J Lipid Res. 1992;33:599–604.
8. Haselwood GAD. The biological importance of bile salts. Amsterdam: North-Holland; 1978.
9. Hammarsten O. über eine neue Gruppe gepaarter Gallensäuren. Z Physiol Chem. 1898;24:322–50.
10. Hoshita T, Kazuno T. Chemistry and metabolism of bile alcohols and higher bile acids. In Paoletti R, Kritchevsky D, editors. Advances in lipid research, Vol. 6. New York: Academic Press; 1968:208–54.
11. Haslewood GAD. Comparative studies of bile salts.5. Bile salts of Crocodylidae. Biochem J. 1952;52:583–7.
12. Williams RT. Species variations in drug biotransformations. In: La Du BN, Mandel HG, Way EL, editors. Fundamentals of drug metabolism and drug disposition. Baltimore: Williams & Wilkins; 1971:187–205.
13. Caldwell J. Conjugation reactions in the metabolism of xenobiotics, In: Arias I, Popper H, Schachter D, Shafritz DA, editors. The liver: biology and pathobiology. New York: Raven Press; 1982:281–295.
14. JI YH, Moog C, Schmitt G, Luu B. Polyoxygenated sterols and triterpenes: chemical structures and biological activities. J Steroid Biochem. 1990;35:741–4.
15. Hofmann AF. Bile acids. In: Arias IM, Boyer JL, Fausto N, Jakoby WB, Schachter D Shafritz DA, editors. The liver: biology and pathobiology. New York: Raven Press; 1994:677–718.
16. Borgström B, Patton JS. Luminal events in gastrointestinal lipid digestion, In: Schultz SG, Field M, Frizzell RA Raunder BB, editors. Handbook of physiology, Vol. 4. Bethesda: American Physiological Society; 1991:475–504.
17. Hofmann AF. Bile acids as drugs: principles, mechanisms of action, and formulations.In: van Berge Henegouwen GP, van Hoek B, de Groote, J, Matern Stockbrugger RW,editors. Bile acids as theraputic drugs. Ital J Gastroenterol. 27;1995 (In press).
18. Cohen BI, Hofmann AF, Mosbach EH *et al.* Differing effects of nor-ursodeoxycholic or ursodeoxycholic acid on hepatic histology and bile acid metabolism in the rabbit. Gastroenterology 1986;91:189–97.
19. Leuschner U. Ursodeoxycholic acid therapy in primary biliary cirrhosis. Scand J Gastroenterol. 1994;29:40–6.
20. Stiehl A. Ursodeoxycholic acid therapy in treatment of primary sclerosing cholangitis. Scand J Gastroenterol. 1994;29:59–61
21. Crombie DL, Hagey LR, Lillienau J, Miyai K, Hofmann AF. Toxicity of orally administered cholyltaurine in the guinea pig: discovery of a rodent that cannot detoxify deoxycholic acid. Gastroenterology. 1992;102:A922(abstract).
22. Hofmann AF, Molino G, Milanese M, Belforte G. Description and simulation of a physiological pharmacokinetic model for the metabolism and enterohepatic circulation of bile acids in man. Cholic acid in healthy man. J Clin Invest. 1983;71;1003–22.
23. Molino G, Hofmann AF, Cravetto C, Belforte G, Bona B. Simulation of the metabolism and enterohepatic circulation of endogenous chenodeoxycholic acid in man using a physiological pharmacokinetic model. Eur J Clin Invest. 1986;16:397–414.
24. Hofmann AF, Cravetto C, Molino G, Belforte G, Bona B. Simulation of the metabolism and enterohepatic circulation of endogenous deoxycholic acid in man using a physiological pharmacokinetic model for bile acid metabolism. Gastroenterology. 1987;93:693–709.
25. Hofmann AF, Hoffman NE. Measurement of bile acid kinetics by isotope dilution in man. Gastroenterology. 1974;67:314–23.

26. Lindstedt S. The turnover of cholic acid in man. Acta Physiol Scand. 1957;40:1–9.
27. Williams RT. Detoxication mechanisms, 2nd edn. London: Chapman & Hall; 1959.
28. Macdonal IA, Bokkenheuser VD, Winter J, McLernon AM, Mosbach EH. Degradation of steroids in the human gut. J Lipid Res. 1983;24:675–700.
29. Hellstrom K, Sjövall J. Turnover of deoxycholic acid in the rabbit. J Lipid Res. 1962;3:397–412.
30. Hagey LR, Odell D, Rossi SS, Crombie DL, Hofmann AF. Biliary bile acid composition of the Physeteridae (sperm whales). Marine Mam Sci. 1993;9:23–33.
31. Strasberg SM, Harvey PR, Hofmann AF. Bile sampling, processing and analysis in clinical studies. Hepatology. 1990;12:176S–180S.
32. Hussaini SH, Kennedy C, Pereira SP, Wass JAH, Dowling RH. Ultrasound-guided percutaneous fine needle puncture of the gallbladder for studies of bile composition. Br J Radiol. 1995;68:271–6.
33. DeMark BR, Everson GT, Klein PD, Showalter RB, Kern F. A method for the accurate measurement of isotope ratios of chenodeoxycholic and cholic acids in serum. J Lipid Res. 1982;23:204–10.
34. Stellaard F, Paumgartner G, van Berge Henegouwen GP, Van Der Werf SD. Determination of deoxycholic acid pool size and input rate using [24-13C] deoxycholic acid and serum sampling. J Lipid Res. 1986;27:1222–5.
35. Mitchell JC, Stone BG, Duane WC. Measurement of bile acid synthesis in man by release of $^{14}CO_2$ from [26-14C] cholesterol: comparison to isotope dilution and assessment of optimum cholesterol specific activity. Lipids. 1992;27:68–71.
36. Bertolotti M, Carulli N, Menozzi D et al. In vivo evaluation of cholesterol 7α-hydroxylation in humans: effect of disease and drug treatment. J Lipid Res 1986;27:1278–86.
37. van der Werf SDJ, Huijbregts AWM, Lamers HLM, van Berge Henegouwen GP, van Tongeren JHM. Age dependent differences in human bile acid metabolism and 7α-dehydroxylation. Eur J Clin Invest. 1981;11:425–31.
38. Berr F, Pratschke E, Fishcer S, Paumgartner G. Disorders of bile acid metabolism in cholesterol gallstone disease. J Clin Invest. 1992;90:859–68.
39. Legrand-Defretin V, Juste C, Corring T, Rerat A. Enterohepatic circulation of bile acids in pigs: diurnal pattern and effect of a re-entrant biliary fistula. Am J Physiol. 1986;250:G295–G301.
40. van Berge Henegouwen GP, Hofmann AF. Systemic spill-over of bile acids. Eur J Clin Invest. 1983;13:433–7.
41. Paumgartner G. Serum bile acids. Physiological determinants and results in liver disease. J Hepatol. 1986;2:291–8.
42. Mallory A, Kern F, Jr Smith J, Savage D. Patterns of bile acids and microflora in the human small intestine. I. Bile acids. Gastroenterology. 1973;64:26–33.
43. Northfield TC, McColl I. Postprandial concentrations of free and conjugated bile acids down the length of the normal human small intestine. Gut. 1973;14:513–18.
44. Angelina B, Einarsson K, Hellstrom K. Evidence for the absorption of bile acids in the proximal small intestine of normo–and hyperlipidaemic subjects. Gut. 1976;17:420–25.
45. Sjövall J, Setchell KDR. Techniques for extraction and group separation of bile acids. In: Setchell KDR, Kritchevsky D, Nair PP, editors. The bile acids: chemistry, physiology, and metabolism, Vol. 4. New York: Plenum Press; 1988:1–42.
46. Nambara T, Goto J. High-performance liquid chromatography. In: Setchell KDR, Kritchevsky D, Nair PP, editors. The bile acids: chemistry, physiology, and metabolism, Vol. 4. New York: Plenum Press; 1988:43–64.
47. Iida T, Tamura T, Matsumoto T, Chang FC. Carbon-13 NMR spectra of hydroxylated bile acid stereoisomers. Org Magn Reson. 1983;21:305–9.
48. Kuroki S, Schteingart CD, Hagey LR et al. Bile salts of the West Indian manatee, Trichechus manatus latirostris: novel bile alcohol sulfates and absence of bile acids. J Lipid Res. 1988;29:509–22.
49. Schteingart CD, Hagey LR, Setchell KDR, Hofmann AF. 5β-Hydroxylation by the liver: identification of 3,5,7-trihydroxy nor-bile acids as new major biotransformation products of 3,7-dihydroxy nor-bile acids in rodents. J Biol Chem. 1993;268:11239–46.
50. Hagey LR, Schteingart CD, Ton-Nu HT, Hofmann AF. Biliary bile acids of fruit pigeons and doves (columbiformes): presence of 1β-hydroxychenodeoxycholic acid and conjugation with glycine as well as taurine. J Lipid Res. 1994;35:2041–8.

51. Lawson AM, Setchell KDR. Mass spectrometry of bile acids. In: Setchell KDR, Kritchevsky D, Nair PP, editors. The bile acids: chemistry, physiology and metabolism, Vol. 4. New York: Plenum Press; 1988:167–268.

52. Iida T, Nambara T, Chang FC. Synthesis of uncommon bile acids. In: Hofmann AF, Paumgartner G, Stiehl A, editors. Bile acids in gastroenterologyy: basic and clinical advances. London: Kluwer;1995:8–26.

53. Russell DW, Setchell KDR. Bile acid biosynthesis. Biochemistry. 1992;31:4737–49.

54. Hagey LR. 1992. Bile acid biodiversity in vertebrates: chemistry and evolutionary implication. Ph.D. thesis, University of California, San Diego, CA: 1–205.

55. Hagey LR. Crombie DL, Espinosa E, Carey MC, Igimi H, Hofmann AF. Ursodeoxycholic acid in the Ursidae: biliary bile acids of bears, pandas, and related carnivores. J Lipid Res. 1993;34:1911–17.

56. Tint GS, Bullock J, Batta AK, Shefer S, Salen G. Ursodeoxycholic acid, 7-ketolithocholic acid, and chenodeoxycholic acid are primary bile acids of the nutria (*Myocastor coypus*). Gastroenterology. 1985;90:702–9.

57. Tint GS, Xu G, Batta AK, Shefer S, Niemann WS. Ursodeoxycholic acid, chenodeoxycholic acid, and 7-ketolithocholic acid are primary bile acids of the guinea pig. J Lipid Res. 1990;31:1301–6.

58. Hagey LR, Takagi K, Schteingart CD, Ton-Nu HT, Hofmann AF. A hydroxy-oxo C24 bile acid with an unsaturated side chain is the predominant biliary bile acid of the mountain paca, a large rodent. Hepatology. 1994;20:A666(abstract).

59. Une M, Hoshita T. Natural occurrence and chemical synthesis of bile alcohols, higher bile acids, and short side chain bile acids. Hiroshima J Med Sci. 1994;43:37–67.

60. Hagey LR, Takagi K, Schteingart CD, Ton-Nu HT, Hofmann AF. C_{24} bile acid reduction into bile alcohols: a novel, ubiquitous minor pathway of cholesterol elimination in vertebrates. Hepatology. 1994;20:A639(abstract).

61. Reichwald-Hacker I. Substrate specificity of enzymes catalyzing the biosynthesis of ether lipids. In: Mangold HK, Paltauf F, editors. Ether lipids: biochemical and biomedical aspects. New York: Academic Press; 1983:129–40.

62. Takagi K, Hagey LR, Schteingart CD, Lance V, Hofmann AF. β-Cyprinol sulfate is a major bile acid in three families of perciform fish. Hepatology. 1994;20:A665(abstract).

63. Hsia SL. Hyocholic acid and muricholic acids. In: Nair PP, Kritchevsky D, editors. The bile acids: chemistry, physiology and metabolism, Vol. 1. New York: Plenum Press, 1971:95–120.

64. Cerrè C, Hagey LR, Schteingart CD, Hofmann AF. Sythesis, natural occurrence, and mass spectrometry of 5β-hydroxy derivatives of natural bile acids. Gastroenterology. 1995 (In press).

65. Hagey LR, Schteingart CD, Ton-Nu H, Rossi SS, Odell D, Hofmann AF. β-Phocaecholic acid in bile: biochemical evidence that the flamingo is related to an ancient goose. Condor. 1990;92:593–7.

66. Pellicciari R, Nataline B, Cecchetti S, Fringuelli R. Reduction of α-diazo-β-hydroxy esters to β-hydroxy esters: application in one of two convergent syntheses of a (22S)-22hydroxy bile acid from fish bile and its (22R)-epimer. J Chem Soc, Perkin Trans. 1985;3:493–7.

67. Hoffman NE, Hofmann AF. Metabolism of steroid and amino acid moieties of conjugated bile acids in man. V. Equations for the perturbed enterohepatic circulation and their application. Gastroenterology. 1977;72:141–8.

68. Hoshita T. Bile alcohols and primitive bile acids. In: Danielsson H, Sjövall J, editors. Sterols and bile acids. Amsteram: Elsevier;1985:279–302.

69. Hagey LR, Schteingart CD, Ton-Nu HT, Hofmann AF. Conjugation of bile acids with *N*-methyl taurine: a new metabolic pathway. Hepatology. 1993;18:305A(abstract).

70. Une M, Got T, Kihira K *el al*. Isolation and identification of bile salts conjugated with cysteinolic acid from the bile of the red seabream, *Pagrosomus major*. J Lipid Res. 1991;32:1619–23.

71. Cowen AE, Korman MG, Hofmann AF, Cass OW. Metabolism of lithocholate in healthy man. I. Biotransformation and biliary excretion of intravenously administered lithocholate, lithocholylglycine, and their sulfates. Gastroenterology. 1975;69:59–66.

72. van Berge Henegouwen GP, Brandt KH, Eyssen H, Parmentier G. Sulphated and unsulphated bile acids in serum, bile, and urine of patients with cholestasis. Gut. 1976;17:861–9.

73. Oude Elferink RPJ, de Haan J, Lambert KJ, Hagey LR, Hofmann AF, Jansen PLM. Selective hepatobiliary transport of nordeoxycholate side chain conjugates in mutant rats with a canalicular transport defect. Hepatology. 1989;9:861–5.

74. Pillot T, Ouzzine M, Fournel-Gigleux S *et al.* Glucuronidation of hyodeoxycholic acid in human liver. Evidence for a selective role of UDP-glucuronosyltransferase 2B4. J Biol Chem. 1993;268:25636–42.

75. Okuda K. Liver mitochondrial P450 involved in cholesterol catabolism and vitamin D activation. J Lipid Res. 1994;35:361–72.

76. Ohshima A, Kuramato T, Hoshita T. Biochemical studies of inherited diseases related to abnormal cholesterol metabolism. I. High-performance liquid chromatographic analysis of bile alcohol glucuronides in cerebrotendinous xanthomatosis. Biol Pharm Bull. 1994;17:721–3.

77. Marschall H-U, Griffiths WJ, Gotze U *et al.* The major metabolites of ursodeoxycholic acid in human urine are conjugated with *N*-acetylglucosamine. Hepatology. 1994;20:845–53.

78. Matern H, Matern S, Gerok W. Isolation and characterization of rat liver microsomal UDP-glucuronosyltransferase activity toward chenodeoxycholic acid and testosterone as a single form of enzyme. J Biol Chem. 1982;257:7422–9.

79. Anwer MS, O'Maille ERL, Hofmann AF, DiPietro RA, Michelotti E. Influence of side-chain charge on hepatic transport of bile acids and bile acid analogues. Am J Physiol. 1985;249:G479–G488.

80. van Berge Henegouwen GP, Hofmann AF. Nocturnal gallbladder storage and emptying in gallstone patients and helathy subjects. Gastroenterology. 1978;75: 879–85.

81. Shindo K, Fukushima K. Deconjugation of bile acids by human intestinal bacteria. Gastroenterol Jpn. 1976;11:167–74.

82. Setchell KDR, Street JM, Sjövall J. Fecal bile acids. In: Setchell KDR, Kritchevsky D, Nair PP, editors. The bile acids: chemistry, physiology and metabolism, Vol. 4. New York: Plenum Press; 1988:441–570.

83. Macdonald IA, Hutchison DM, Forrest TP, Bokkenheuser VD, Winter J, Holdeman LV. Metabolism of primary bile acids by *Clostridium perfringens*. J Steroid Biochem. 1983;18:97–104.

84. Zhang R, Barnes S, Diasio RB. Differential intestinal deconjugation of taurine and glycine bile acid *N*-acyl amidates in rats. Am J Physiol. 1992;262:G351–8.

85. Hepner GW, Hofmann AF, Thomas PJ. Metabolism of steroid and amino acid moieties of conjugated bile acids in man. I. Cholylglycine. J Clin Invest. 1972;51:1889–97.

86. Hepner GW, Sturman JA, Hofmann AF, Thomas PJ. Metabolism of steroid and amino acid moieties of conjugated bile acids in man. III. Cholyltaurine (taurocholic acid). J Clin Invest. 1973;52:433–40.

87. Schmassmann A, Hofmann AF, Angellotti MA *et al.* Prevention of ursodeoxycholate hepatotoxicity in the rabbit by conjugation with *N*-methyl amino acids. Hepatology. 1990;11:989–96.

88. Schmassmann A, Fehr HF, Locher J *et al.* Cholylsarcosine, a new bile acid analogue: metabolism and effect on biliary secretion in humans. Gastroenterolgy. 1993;104:1171–81.

89. Kimura M, Hatono S, Une M, Fukuoka C, Kuramato T, Hoshita T. Synthesis, intestinal absorption, and metabolism of sarcosine conjugated ursodeoxycholic acid. Steroids. 1984;43:677–87.

90. Cowen AE, Korman MG, Hofmann AF, Cass OW, Coffin SB. Metabolism of lithocholate in healthy man. II. Enterohepatic circulation. Gastroenterology. 1975;69:67–76.

91. Huijghebaert S, Parmentier G, Eyssen H. Specificity of bile salt sulfatase activity in man, mouse and rat intestinal microflora. J Steroid Biochem. 1984;20:907–12.

92. Hylemon PB. Metabolism of bile acids in intestinal microflora. In: Danielsson H, Sjövall J, editors. Sterols and bile acids. Amsterdam: Elsevier, 1985;331–43.

93. Mallonee DH, White WB, Hylemon PB. Cloning and sequencing of a bile acid-inducible operon from *Eubacterium* sp. strain VP1 12708. J Bacteriol. 1990;172:7011–19.

94. Coleman JP, White WB, Egestad B, Sjövall J, Hylemon PB. Biosynthesis of a novel bile acid nucleotide and mechanism of 7 alpha-dehydroxylation by an intestinal *Eubacterium* species. J Biol Chem. 1987;262:4701–7.

95. Mikami T, Kihira K, Ikawa S *et al.* Metabolism of sulfonate analogs of ursodeoxycholic acid and their effects on biliary bile acid composition in hamsters. J Lipid Res. 1993;34:429–35.

96. Lindqvist A, Midtvedt T, Skrede S, Sjövall J. Effect of bile alcohols on the microbial 7α-dehydroxylation of chenodeoxycholic acid. Microb Ecol Health Dis. 1990;3:25–32.

97. Bokkenheuser V, Hoshita T, Mosbach EH. Bacterial 7α-dehydroxylation of cholic acid and allocholic acid. J Lipid Res. 1969;10:421–6.

98. Tint GS, Batta AK, Dayal B, Kovell N, Shefer S, Salen G. Metabolism of ursocholic acid in humans: conversion of ursocholic acid to deoxycholic acid. Hepatology. 1992;15:645–50.

99. Samuelsson B. Studies on the mechanism of the formation of hyodeoxycholic acid in the pig. Arkh Kemi. 1960;15:425–32.

100. Miki S, Mosbach EH, Cohen BI *et al.* Metabolism of β-muricholic acid in the hamster and prairie dog. J Lipid Res. 1993;34:1709–16.

101. Sacquet E, Parquet M, Riottot M, Raizman A, Nordlinger B, Infante R. Metabolism of β-muricholic acid in man. Steroids. 1985;45:411–26.

102. Setoguchi T, Higashi S, Tateno S, Yahiro K, Katsuki T. Epimerization of the four 3,7-dihydroxy bile acid epimers by human fecal microorganisms in anaerobic mixed cultures and in feces. J Lipid Res. 1984;25:1246–56.

103. Macdonald IA, Rochon YP, Hutchison DM, Holdeman LV. Formation of ursodeoxycholic acid from chenodeoxycholic acid by a 7 beta-hydroxysteroid dehydrogenase-elaborating *Eubacterium aerofaciens* strain cocultured with 7α-hydroxysteroid dehydrogenase-elaborating organisms. Appl Environ Microbiol. 1982;44:1187–95.

104. Hirano S, Masuda N, Oda H. *In vitro* transformation of chenodeoxycholic acid and ursodeoxycholic acid by human intestinal flora, with particular reference to the mutual conversion between the two bile acids. J Lipid Res. 1981;22:735–43.

105. Hardison WGM. Hepatic taurine concentration and dietary taurine as regulators of bile acid conjugation with taurine. Gastroenterology. 1978;75:71–5.

106. Clerici C, Gurantz D, Hagey LR, Schteingart CD, Hofmann AF. Nor-lithocholate's choleretic effect depends on species specific hepatic biotransformation. Hepatology. 1986;6:1143(abstract).

107. Gadacz TR, Allan RN, Mack E, Hofmann AF. Impaired lithocholate sulfation in the rhesus monkey: a possible mechanism for chenodeoxycholate toxicity. Gastroenterology. 1976;70:1125–9.

108. Palmer RH. Bile acids, liver injury, and liver disease. Arch Intern Med. 1972;130:606–17.

109. Palmer RH. Toxic effects of lithocholate on the liver and biliary tree, In: Taylor W, editor. The hepatobiliary system: fundamental and pathological mechanism. New York: Plenum Press, 1976:227–40.

110. Matern S, Sjövall J, Pomare EW, Heaton KW, Low-Beer TS. Metabolism of deoxycholic acid in man. Med Biol. 1975;53:107–13.

111. Hofmann AF, Grundy SM, Lachin JM *et al.* Pretreatment biliary lipid composition in white patients with radiolucent gallstones in the National Cooperative Gallstone Study. Gastroenterology. 1982;83:738–52.

112. Clayton LM, Gurantz D, Hofmann AF, Hagey LR, Schteingart CD. Role of bile acid conjugation in hepatic transport of dihydroxy bile acids. J Pharmacol Exp Ther. 1989;248:1130–7.

113. Bergström S, Danielsson H, Kazuno T. Bile acids and steroids: the metabolism of bile acids in python and constrictor snakes. J Biol Chem. 1960;235:983–88.

114. Murakami K, Okuda K. Purification and characterization of taurodeoxycholate 7α-monooxygenase in rat liver. J Biol Chem. 1981;256:8658–62.

115. Ananthanarayanan M, Von Dippe P, Levy D. Identification of the hepatocyte Na+-dependent bile acid transport protein using monoclonal antibodies. J Biol Chem. 1988;263:8338–43.

116. Takikawa H, Stolz A, Kuroki S, Kaplowitz N. Oxidation and reduction of bile acid precursors by rat hepatic 3α-hydroxysteroid dehydrogenase and inhibition by bile acids and indomethacin. Biochim Biophys Acta. 1990;1043:153–6.

117. Stolz A, Rahimi-Kiani M, Ameis D, Chan E, Ronk M, Shively JE. Molecular structure of rat hepatic 3 alpha-hydroxysteroid dehydrogenase. A member of the oxidoreductase gene family. J Biol Chem. 1991;266:15253–7.

118. Cantafora A, Alavaro D, Attili AF *et al.* Hepatic 3α-dehydrogenation and 7α-hydroxylation of deoxycholic acid in the guinea-pig. Comp Biochem Physiol [B]. 1986;85:805–10.

119. Shefer S, Salen G, Hauser S, Dayal B, Batta AK. Metabolism of iso-bile acids in the rat. J Biol Chem. 1982;257:1401–6.

120. Marcus SN, Schteingart CD, Marquez ML *et al.* Active absorption of conjugated bile acids *in vivo*. Kinetic parameters and molecular specificity of the ileal transport system in the rat. Gastroenterology. 1991;100:212–21.

121. Nakagaki M, Danzinger RG, Hofmann AF, DiPietro RA. Biliary secretion and hepatic metabolism of taurine conjugated 7α-hydroxy and 7β-hydroxy bile acids in the dog: defective hepatic transport and bile hyposecretion. Gastroenterolgoy. 1984;87:647–59.

122. Fromm H, Carlson GL, Hofmann AF, Farivar S, Amin P. Metabolism in man of 7-ketolithocholic acid: precursor of cheno-and ursodeoxycholic acids. Am J Physiol. 1980;239:G161–6.

123. Yamashita H, Setchell KDR. Metabolism and effect of 7-oxo-lithocholic acid 3-sulfate on bile flow and biliary lipid secretion in rats. Hepatology. 1994;20:663–71.

124. Batta AK, Salen G, Shefer S, Tint GS, Dayal B. The effect of tauroursodeoxycholic acid and taurine supplementation on biliary bile acid composition. Hepatology. 1982;2:811–16.

125. Hardison WGM, Grundy SM. Effect of ursodeoxycholate and its taurine conjugate on bile acid synthesis and cholesterol absorption. Gastroenterology. 1984;87:130–5.

126. Furio L, Tomaiuolo P, Gatta R, Tomaiuolo M. Treatment of virus-associated liver cirrhosis with tauroursodeoxycholic acid–evaluation of cytolysis and cholestasis indexes and selected immunologic variables. Curr Therap Res. 1994;55:1355–62.

127. Dimario F, Delfavero G, Scalon P, Meggiato T. Tauroursodeoxycholic acid in the treatment of biliary dyspepsia. Adv Therapy. 1994;11:262–8.

128. Portincasa P, Palmieri V, Doronzo F *et al*. Effect of tauroursodeoxycholic acid on serum liver enzymes and dyspeptic symptoms in patients with chronic active hepatitis. Curr Therap Res. 1993;53:521–32.

129. Notarbartolo A, Montalto G, Soresi M, Bascone F. Tauroursodeoxycholic acid in patients with chronic hepatitis-C: effect on serum levels of transaminases and γ-glutamyl transpeptidase. Adv Therapy. 1994;11:34–41.

130. Hofmann AF. The cholehepatic circulation of unconjugated bile acids: an update, In: Paumgartner G, Stiehl A, Gerok W, editors. Bile acids and the hepatobiliary system. Boston: Kluwer; 1993:143–60.

131. Hofmann AF. Enterohepatic circulation of bile acids. In: Schultz SG, editors. Handbook of physiology. Section on the gastrointestinal system. Bethesda: American Physiological Society, 1989:567–96.

132. Nakatomi F, Kihira K, Kuramoto T, Hoshita T. Intestinal absorption and metabolism of norcholic acid in rats. J Pharmacobiodyn. 1985;8:557–63.

133. Borgström B, Barrowman J, Krabisch L, Lindstrom M, Lillienau J. Effects of cholic acid, 7β-hydroxy and 12β-hydroxy isocholic acid on bile flow, lipid secretion and bile acid synthesis in the rat. Scand J Clin Lab Invest. 1986;46:167–75.

134. Thistle JL, Schoenfield LJ. Induced alterations in composition of bile of persons having cholelithiasis. Gastroenterology. 1971;61:488–96.

135. Balducci R, Road A, Pearlman RS. A theoretical model for the critical micelle concentration of bile salts. J Solution Chem. 1989;18:355–68.

136. Hofmann AF, Mekhjian HS. Bile acids and the intestinal absorption of fat and electrolytes in health and disease. In: Nair PP, Kritchevsky D, editors. The bile acids: chemistry, physiology, and metabolism, Vol II. New York: Plenum Press; 1973:103–52.

137. Schiff ER, Small NC, Dietschy JM. Characterization of the kinetics of the passive and active transport mechanisms for bile acid absorption in the small intestine and colon of the rat. J Clin Invest. 1972;51:1351–62.

138. Dupas JL, Hofmann AF. Passive jejunal absorption of bile acids *in vivo*: structure–activity relationships and rate limiting steps. Gastroenterology. 1984;86:1067.

139. Cabral DJ, small DM, Lilly HS, Hamilton JA. Transbilayer movement of bile acids in model membranes. Biochemistry. 1987;26:1801–4.

140. Merrill JR, Peng Y, Schteingart CD *et al*. Ecological and metabolic properties of phocaecholic acid, a natural α-hydroxy bile acid present in wading birds. Gastroenterology. 1991;100:A835.

141. Hofmann AF, Mysels KJ. Bile acid solubility and precipitation *in vitro* and *in vivo*: the role of conjugation, pH, and Ca^{++} ions. J Lipid Res. 1992;33:617–26.

142. Huijghebaert SM, Hofmann AF. Pancreatic carboxypeptidase hydrolysis of bile acid-amino acid conjugates: selective resistance of glycine and taurine amidates. Gastroenterology. 1986;90:306–15.

2
Role of alternative pathways of bile acid biosynthesis in liver disease

J. SJÖVALL

INTRODUCTION

The biosynthesis of bile acids from cholesterol involves at least 15 enzymes which are present in the endoplasmic reticulum, the mitochondria, the peroxisomes or the cytosol[1]. Many of the enzymes have a dual subcellular localization and some of the reactions can be catalysed by alternative enzymes. For this reason there are many possible reaction sequences that can lead to bile acids and, if an enzyme is lacking, alternative end-products are produced which in turn may undergo their own metabolism, e.g. hydroxylation, oxidoreduction or conjugation.

It is well known that many bile acids are cytotoxic and cause cholestasis [2]. Hydrophobicity of a bile acid is positively correlated to its cytotoxicity[3]. The question of whether there are structure-specific interactions between bile acids and cellular components is more difficult to answer. In recent years inborn and secondary enzyme deficiencies have been found which lead to formation of structurally very specific bile acids and at the same time cholestatic liver disease[4–6]. One could therefore speculate that the numerous pathways for bile acid biosynthesis that are open could sometimes lead to elevated levels of intermediates which specifically disturb some function of the hepatocyte.

PATHWAYS OF BILE ACID BIOSYNTHESIS

It is now well established that bile acid biosynthesis can start either in the endoplasmic reticulum with 7α-hydroxylation of cholesterol or in the mitochondria with 27-hydroxylation, the latter leading preferentially to chenodeoxycholic acid[7–9]. Cholesterol 7α-hydroxylase is subject to feedback regulation by bile acids and a rate-limiting step for this pathway[1]. It was recently shown that the 27-hydroxylase is also regulated in a similar way, although to a lesser degree[10,11]. The alternative start of bile acid synthesis in two different compartments suggests that newly synthesized and preformed cholesterol may be differently channelled to cholic and chenodeoxycholic acid. In addition to the subcellular compartmentation, the cholesterol 7α-hydroxylase is exclusively, and the sterol 27-hydroxylase preferentially, expressed in the perivenous hepatocytes. The expression in the periportal cells increases when the enterohepatic circulation is interrupted[12]. This distribution opens further possibilities for selective biological effects of intermediates in bile acid biosynthesis.

When 27-hydroxylation is the first reaction, the subsequent 7α-hydroxylation is catalysed by an enzyme different from cholesterol 7α-hydroxylase[13–17]. This enzyme does not seem to be feedback-regulated, but it has not yet been purified or a cDNA cloned. A similar 7α-hydroxylation is expressed in human diploid fibroblasts[18], and we later found it in brain microsomes[19]. Since fibroblasts can also oxidize the 3β- and 27-hydroxy groups[1] they can form C_{27} intermediates which can be converted to normal bile acids in the liver. The pathophysiological implications of this finding are not known, but work in collaboration with Björkhem's group indicates some importance of an extrahepatic bile acid formation *in vivo*[20].

The side-chain oxidation to C_{24} bile acids can occur at any stage of the synthesis from 3β-hydroxy-5-cholestenoic acid and onwards. It normally takes place in the peroxisomes[21]. It is interesting that disorders of the side-chain degradation, e.g. cerebrotendinous xanthomatosis (CTX) with lack of 27-hydroxylase, do not have liver disease as a prominent feature. Perhaps this is not surprising, since bile alcohols and C_{27} bile acids are the functional bile salts in primitive species. It should also be remembered that CTX patients make cholic acid via the alternative 25-hydroxylation pathway[21], and this may be enough to drive bile acid-dependent bile flow.

The first structural rearrangements of the A/B rings are catalysed by the specific 3β-hydroxy-Δ^5-C_{27}-steroid dehydrogenase/isomerase and then by a 3-oxo-Δ^4-steroid 5β-reductase[1]. The former requires the presence of a 7α-hydroxy group and the reaction can take place once this group has been introduced. The 5β-reductase has been purified and a cDNA cloned[22,23]. In the pathway to cholic acid in humans a 12α-hydroxy group is introduced into a substrate with a $3\beta,7\alpha$-dihydroxy-Δ^5 or 7α-hydroxy-3-oxo-Δ^4 structure.

DEFICIENCIES OF 3β-HYDROXY-Δ^5-C_{27}-STEROID DEHYDROGENASE/ISOMERASE (3β-C_{27}-HSDH) AND 3-OXO-Δ^4-STEROID 5β-REDUCTASE (5β-RED)

Absence of any one of these two enzymes leads to cholestatic liver disease[4–6,24–26]. Because of the low specificity of many of the enzymes used in bile acid synthesis, patients with these deficiencies still make C_{24} bile acids but with the incompletely transformed A/B ring structures. However, they also excrete compounds formed along alternative metabolic pathways. For example, the side-chain degradation may not be as effective as normally. Thus, patients with 3β-C_{27}-HSDH deficiency excrete sulphated bile alcohols in bile[27], and patients with 5β-Red deficiency often have glucuronidated C_{27}-bile alcohols in urine[28]. In both cases the incompletely transformed A/B-rings are the same in the bile alcohols as in the corresponding bile acids. In 5β-Red deficiency a 5α-reductase may take over and reduce some of the Δ^4 acids to allo bile acids[6]. This is apparently not enough to produce a bile flow.

Both these diseases have one factor in common: the patients do not excrete the abnormal bile acids in bile. This indicates a bile acid transport problem. However, the patients with 3β-C_{27}-HSDH deficiency excrete their acids together with an array of bile alcohols and C_{27} acids as sulphates in bile. We have assumed that this excretion does not use the normal bile acid transporter but rather the multispecific organic anion transporter[29]. The biliary excretion of the sulphates provides the intestinal bacteria with substrates for hydrolysis by sulphatase(s) and oxidation by the microbial 3β-hydroxysteroid dehydrogenase[30]. Thus, the intestinal flora and the liver in symbiosis are able to make some normal bile acids and this may explain why some patients survive for many years without treatment. The same option is not open for patients with 5β-Red deficiency since their pathological bile acids have no 3-hydroxy group for sulphation and the non-sulphated bile acids are not excreted in bile.

Since there was an apparent defect in the biliary secretion of bile acids with an abnormal A/B-ring structure and conformation, a collaborative project was initiated to see if these acids could be transported by the ATP-dependent canalicular bile acid transport system[29]. Labelled and unlabelled taurine conjugates were prepared as water-soluble analogues of $3\beta,7\alpha$-dihyroxy-5-cholenoic and 7α-hydroxy-3-oxo-4-cholenoic acids. These compounds did not exhibit ATP-dependent transport in canilicular plasma membrane vesicles. In addition, they strongly inhibited the transport of cholyltaurine[31]. These results provide a probable explanation for the intrahepatic cholestasis in patients lacking 3β-C_{27}-HSDH or 5β-Red. Administration of normal bile acids provides the transport system with substrate that can be transported and produce a bile acid-dependent bile flow. In addition it may suppress 7α-hydroxylation and 27-hydroxylation so that the formation of inhibitory endogenous bile acids is reduced (see chapter 4).

Many liver diseases are accompanied by a secondary deficiency of 5β-Red[5,24]. This might be important for the progression of liver damage. When the level of enzyme has decreased to a point that makes 5β-reduction a rate-limiting step, 7α-hydroxy-3-oxo-4-cholenoic acid is formed and can inhibit canalicular secretion of normal bile acids. This may lead to retention of cytotoxic bile acids leading to further hepatocyte damage and decrease of 5β-Red. This vicious circle is illustrated in Fig.1. Supporting this hypothesis, oral administration of chenodeoxycholic acid to a patient with 5β-Red deficiency aggravated the cholestasis and liver function, which returned to pretreatment levels when chenodeoxycholic acid was withdrawn[32]. Cholic acid is much less toxic and has been used in combination with ursodeoxycholic acid for successful treatment of several cases of 5β-Red deficiency. One can speculate about the potential importance of 12α-hydroxylation as a protective mechanism in cases of 5β-Red deficiency, and it would be important to investigate whether $7\alpha,12\alpha$-dihydroxy-3-oxo-4-cholenoic acid inhibits canalicular bile acid transport as strongly as the analogue without the 12α-hydroxy group. The ratio of cholic to chenodeoxycholic acid is known to decrease with advancing liver disease. This could indicate a change of biosynthetic pathway or a loss of 12α-hydroxylase activity. The most serious cases of 5β-Red described appeared to have chenodeoxycholic acid in small amounts as the only normal bile acid[6,25,28].

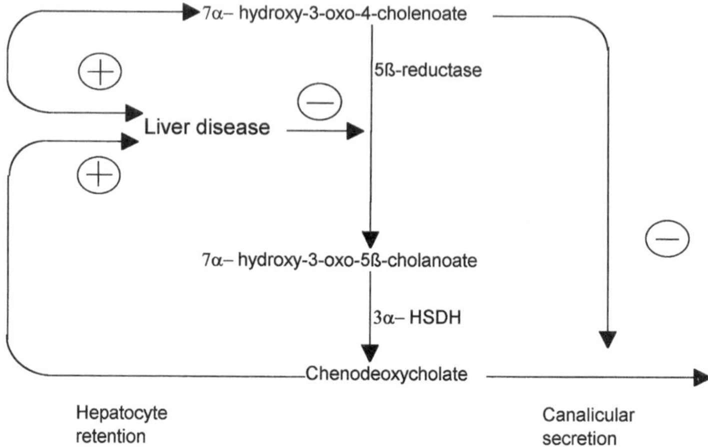

Fig. 1 Proposed vicious circle creating progressive cholestatic liver disease in conditions with primary or secondary 3-oxo-Δ^4-steroid 5β-reductase deficiency

ETHANOL AND BILE ACID BIOSYNTHESIS

Since ethanol oxidation affects oxidoreductions in hepatic steroid metabolism[33], we studied whether it would also affect reactions in bile acid biosynthesis catalysed by NAD$^+$-or NADP$^+$-dependent dehydrogenases. While acute redox effects were not found, the plasma levels of 7α-hydroxycholesterol and 7α-hydroxy-4-cholesten-3-one increased 5–15-fold at 3–4 h after ingestion of a small dose of alcohol[34]. The mechanism behind this effect has not yet been elucidated, but the increased concentrations of the steroids may reflect a stimulation of bile acid synthesis through upregulation of cholesterol 7α-hydroxylase[35]. This would be of interest with regard to the reduced risks of cardiovascular and gallstone disease following small daily doses of alcohol.

The increased levels of 7α-hydroxy-4-cholesten-3-one are of interest in relation to alcoholic liver disease. Thus, 4,6-cholestadien-3-one was identified in the livers of alcoholics[36]. This compound can be formed by 7α-dehydroxylation of 7α-hydroxy-4-cholesten-3-one in the liver (see ref. 26). In view of the hepatotoxic effects of bile acids with a 3-oxo-Δ^4 structure discussed above, a pathophysiological role of neutral intermediates with this structure in alcohol-induced liver disease cannot be excluded. Acetaldehyde formed during the metabolism of alcohol was recently reported to form an adduct with 5β-Red[37]. If this results in a lower activity of the enzyme it could represent a mechanism by which intermediates with a 7α-hydroxy-3-oxo-Δ^4 structure could accumulate during alcohol metabolism. It is also of interest that such intermediates are potent suppressors of the activity of 3-hydroxy-3-methylglutaryl-coenzyme A reductase[38]. This provides another hypothetical link between ethanol metabolism and cholesterol–bile acid metabolism that deserves further studies.

INTRAHEPATIC CHOLESTASIS OF PREGNANCY (ICP)

Although the aetiology is unknown, the cholestasis in this disease is thought to be induced by some steroid hormonal factor. Bile acids in plasma are always increased in ICP, as are a number of sulphated progesterone metabolites[39]. Although the latter are also present in normal pregnancy, and increase markedly during the latter half of pregnancy[40], both the absolute and relative levels of the different steroid sulphate isomers are changed in patients with ICP. It is an important question whether the changes of steroid sulphate levels and patterns are of aetiological importance or merely reflect insufficient biliary excretion due to cholestasis induced by unknown factors.

Ursodeoxycholic acid therapy was recently shown to be very effective in most cases with ICP[41]. Pruritus and serum levels of bile acids and transaminase improved significantly during this treatment. We are therefore performing a comprehensive analytical study of steroids and bile acids in these patients before and during therapy with ursodeoxycholic acid. We have hypothesized that the large load of progesterone (250–300 mg/24 h in late pregnancy) might compete with intermediates in bile acid biosynthesis as substrate for 5β-reductase and 3α-hydroxysteroid dehydrogenase, resulting in formation of cholestatic compounds in certain individuals. So far the studies have revealed that ursodeoxycholic acid lowers not only bile acids but also the elevated levels of steroid mono- and disulphates in plasma[42]. These results are compatible with an effect of ursodeoxycholic acid on the biliary secretion of the steroid sulphates, possibly due to the stimulation of vesicular exocytosis[43]. Whether or not there is also a change of hepatic progesterone metabolism related to the change of steroid sulphate and bile acid secretion remains to be studied.

SUMMARY

Decreased activities or complete lack of certain enzymes in bile acid biosynthesis can lead to elevated levels of intermediates or side-products in alternative pathways which damage the hepatocyte or its secretory functions. It will be of interest to study whether the enzymes exhibit a polymorphism that makes some individuals more sensitive than others to external interferences with the pathways of bile acid biosynthesis leading to accumulation of hepatotoxic compounds.

References

1. Russell DW, Setchell KDR. Bile acid biosynthesis. Biochemistry. 1992;31:4737–49.
2. Heaton KW. Bile salts in health and disease. Edinburgh and London: Churchill Livingstone; 1972.
3. Heuman DM. Hepatoprotective properties of ursodeoxycholic acid. Gastroenterology. 1993;104:1865–70.
4. Clayton PT, Leonard JV, Lawson AM *et al.* Familial giant cell hepatitis associated with synthesis of $3\beta,7\alpha$-dihydroxy-and $3\beta,7\alpha,12\alpha$-trihydroxy-5-cholenoic acids. J Clin Invest. 1987;79:1031–8.
5. Clayton PT, Patel E, Lawson AM *et al.* 3-Oxo-Δ^4 bile acids in liver disease. Lancet. 1988;2:1283–4.
6. Setchell KDR, Suchy FJ, Welsh MB, Zimmer-Nechemias L, Heubi J, Balistreri WF. Δ-3-Oxosteroid 5β-reductase deficiency described in identical twins with neonatal hepatitis. J Clin Invest. 1988;82:2148–57.

7. Axelson M, Sjövall J. Potential bile acid precursors in plasma – possible indicators of biosynthetic pathways to cholic and chenodeoxycholic acids in man. J Steroid Biochem. 1990;36:631–40.

8. Princen HMG, Meijer P, Wolthers BG, Vonk RJ, Kuipers F. Cyclosporin A blocks bile acid synthesis in cultured hepatocytes by specific inhibition of chenodeoxycholic acid synthesis. Biochem J. 1991;275:501–5.

9. Javitt NB. Bile acid synthesis from cholesterol: regulatory and auxiliary pathways. FASEB J. 1994;8:1308–11.

10. Twisk J, de Wit ECM, Princen HMG. Suppression of sterol 27-hydroxylase mRNA and transcriptional activity by bile acids in cultured rat hepatocytes. XXIII International Bile Acid Meeting, Falk Symposium No. 80;30 Sept–2 Nov 1994; San Diego, abstract no. 81.

11. Vlahcevic ZR, Jairath SK, Heuman DM, Hylemon PB, Pandak WM. Coordinate regulation of sterol 27-hydroxylase and cholesterol 7α-hydroxylase by bile acid feedback control. XIII International Bile Acid Meeting, Falk Symposium No. 80;30 Sept–2 Oct 1994; San Diego, abstract no. 17.

12. Princen HMG, Twisk J, Hoekman MFM et al. Heterogeneous distribution of cholesterol 7α-hydroxylase and sterol 27-hydroxylase in the rat liver acinus is regulated at the mRNA and transcriptional level. XIII International Bile Acid Meeting, Falk Symposium No. 80;30 Sept–20 Oct 1994; San Diego, abstract no. 13.

13. Axelson M, Shoda J, Sjövall J, Toll A, Wikvall K. Cholesterol is converted to 7α-hydroxy-3-oxo-4-cholestenoic acid in liver mitochondria. J Biol Chem. 1992;267:1701–4.

14. Toll A, Shoda J, Axelson M, Sjövall J, Wikvall K. 7α-Hydroxylation of 26-hydroxycholesterol, 3β-hydroxy-5-cholestenoic acid and 3β-hydroxy-5-cholenoic acid by cytochrome P-450 in pig liver microsomes. FEBS Lett. 1992;296:73–6.

15. Shoda J, Toll A, Axelson M, Pieper F, Wikvall K, Sjövall J. Formation of 7α- and 7β-hydroxylated bile acid precursors from 27-hydroxycholesterol in human liver microsomes and mitochondria. Hepatology. 1993;17:395–403.

16. Björkhem I, Nyberg B, Einarsson K. 7α-Hydroxylation of 27-hydroxycholesterol in human liver microsomes. Biochim Biophys Acta. 1992;1128:73–6.

17. Martin KO, Budai K, Javitt NB. Cholesterol and 27-hydroxycholesterol 7α-hydroxylation: evidence for two different enzymes. J Lipid Res. 1993;34:581–8.

18. Zhang J, Larsson O, Sjövall J. 7α-Hydroxylation of 25-hydroxycholesterol and 27-hydroxycholesterol in human fibroblasts. Biochim Biophys Acta. 1995;1256:353–9.

19. Zhang J, Akwa Y, Baulieu E-E, Sjövall J. 7α-Hydroxylation of 27-hydroxycholesterol in rat brain microsomes. CR Acad Sci Paris. 1995;318:345–9.

20. Lund E, Andersson O, Zhang J et al. Importance of a novel oxidative mechanism for elimination of intracellular cholesterol in man. 1995 (submitted).

21. Björkhem I. Mechanism of degradation of the steroid side chain in the formation of bile acids. J Lipid Res. 1992;33:455–71.

22. Onishi Y, Noshiro M, Shimosato T, Okuda K. Molecular cloning and sequence analysis of cDNA encoding Δ^4-3-ketosteroid 5β-reductase of rat liver. FEBS Lett. 1991;283:215–18.

23. Kondo K-H, Kai M-H, Setoguchi Y et al. Cloning and expression of cDNA of human Δ^4-3-oxosteroid 5β-reductase and substrate specificity of the expressed enzyme. Eur J Biochem. 1994;219:357–63.

24. Clayton PT. Inborn errors of bile acid metabolism. J Inher Metab Dis. 1991;14:478–96.

25. Setchell KDR, O'Connell NC. Inborn errors of bile acid metabolism. In: Suchy FJ, editor. Liver disease in children. St Louis: Mosby; 1994:835–51.

26. Björkhem I, Muri-Boberg K. Inborn errors in bile acid biosynthesis and storage of sterols other than cholesterol. In: Scriver CR, Beaudet AL, Sly WS, Valle D, editors. The metabolic basis of inherited diseases, 7th edn. New York: McGraw-Hill; 1994:2073–100.

27. Ichimiya H, Egestad B, Nazer H, Baginski ES, Clayton PT, Sjövall J. Bile acids and bile alcohols in a child with hepatic 3β-hydroxy-Δ^5-C_{27}-steroid dehydrogenase deficiency: effects of chenodeoxycholic acid treatment. J Lipid Res. 1991;32:829–41.

28. Sjövall J. Mass spectrometry in studies of inherited and acquired diseases of bile acid synthesis and metabolism. In: Matsumoto I, Kuhara T, Mamer OA, Sweetman L, Calderhead RG, editors. Advances in chemical diagnosis and treatment of metabolic diseases, Vol. 2. Kanazawa Medical University Press; 1995:107–22.

29. Meier PJ. Molecular mechanisms of bile acid transport in hepatocytes. In: van Berge Henegouwen GP, van Hoek B, de Groote J, Matern S, Stockbrügger RW, editors. Cholestatic liver diseases. Dordrecht/Boston/London: Kluwer; 1994:55–61

30. Hylemon PB. Metabolism of bile acids in intestinal microflora. In: Danielsson H, Sjövall J, editors. Sterols and bile acids. Amsterdam: Elsevier; 1985:331–43.

31. Stieger B, Zhang J, O'Neill B, Sjövall J, Meier PJ. Transport of taurine conjugates of 7α-hydroxy-3-oxo-4-cholenoic acid and $3\beta,7\alpha$-dihydroxy-5-cholenoic acid in rat liver plasma membrane vesicles. In: van Berge Henegouwen GP, van Hoek B, de Groote J, Matern S, Stockbrügger RW, editors. Cholestatic liver diseases. Dordrecht/Boston/London: Kluwer; 1994:82–7.

32. Ichimiya H, Nazer H, Gunasekaran T, Clayton P, Sjövall J. Treatment of chronic liver disease caused by 3β-hydroxy-Δ^5-C_{27}-steroid dehydrogenase deficiency with chenodeoxycholic acid. Arch Dis Childh. 1990;65:1121–4.

33. Andersson S, Cronholm T, Sjövall J. Redox effects of ethanol on steroid metabolism. Alcohol Clin Exp Res. 1986;10:55S–63S.

34. Axelson M, Mörk B, Sjövall J. Ethanol has an acute effect on bile acid biosynthesis in man. FEBS Lett. 1991;281:155–9.

35. Axelson M, Björkhem I, Reihner E, Einarsson K. The plasma level of 7α-hydroxy-4-cholesten-3-one reflects the activity of hepatic cholesterol 7α-hydroxylase in man. FEBS Lett. 1991;284:216–18.

36. Ryzlak MT, Fales HM, Russell WL, Schaffner CP. Oxysterols and alcoholic liver disease. Alcohol Clin Exp Res. 1990;14:490–5.

37. Zhu Y, Crabb DW, Lin RC. Identification of the 37 kD rat liver protein which forms acetaldehyde adduct *in vivo* as Δ^4-3-ketosteroid 5β-reductase by molecular cloning and sequencing. Hepatology. 1994;20:269A.

38. Axelson M, Larsson O, Zhang J, Shoda J, Sjövall J. Structural specificity in the suppression of HMG-CoA reductase in human fibroblasts by intermediates in bile acid biosynthesis. J Lipid Res. 1995;36:290–8.

39. Sjövall J, Sjövall K. Steroid sulphates in plasma from pregnant women with pruritus and elevated plasma bile acid levels. Ann Clin Res. 1970;2:321–37.

40. Sjövall K. Gas chromatographic determination of steroid sulphates in plasma during pregnancy. Ann Clin Res. 1970;2:393–408.

41. Palma J, Reyes H, Ribalta J et al. Effects of ursodeoxycholic acid in patients with intrahepatic cholestasis of pregnancy. Hepatology. 1992;15:1043–7.

42. Meng LJ, Reyes H, Palma J, Hernandez I, Ribalta J, Sjövall J. Profiles of steroids and bile acids in plasma of patients with intrahepatic cholestasis of pregnancy – effect of ursodeoxycholic acid therapy. In: van Berge Henegouwen GP, van Hoek B, de Groote J, Matern S, Stockbrügger RW, editors. Cholestatic liver diseases. Dordrecht/Boston/London: Kluwer; 1994:45–9.

43. Beuers U, Nathanson MH, Isales CM, Boyer JL. Tauroursodeoxycholic acid stimulates hepatocellular exocytosis and mobilizes extracellular Ca^{++} mechanisms defective in cholestasis. J Clin Invest. 1993;92:2984–93.

3
Regulation of bile acid synthesis

Z. R. VLAHCEVIC, W. M. PANDAK and P. B. HYLEMON

Two primary bile acids, cholic and chenodeoxycholic, are end-products of cholesterol degradation, a process which takes place exclusively in the liver. The synthesis of bile acids from cholesterol is important for a number of reasons: (a) approximately 50% of daily cholesterol elimination from the body occurs via its degradation to bile acids; (b) bile acid synthesis replenishes daily bile acid faecal losses, thus maintaining the size of the circulating bile acid pool size; (c) bile acids in the enterohepatic circulation perform a number of important physiological functions, including solubilization of other lipids in bile, solubilization of digested fat in the intestine, and intestinal solubilization of calcium and iron; and (d) bile acids play an important role in the mobilization and transfer of hepatic cholesterol and phospholipids, destined for the secretion into the bile[1]. Because of their detergent properties hydrophobic bile acids can be damaging to hepatic membranes; they have been postulated to cause and/or perpetuate liver injury in cholestatic disorders. In cholestatic liver diseases in which there is impairment of bile flow, bile acids accumulate in the liver, possibly contributing to the liver injury. Conversely, hydrophilic bile acids have been shown to be hepatoprotective against the detergent action of hydrophobic bile acids[2,3]. For example, administration of ursodeoxycholic acid, a hydrophilic bile acid, results in the improvement of liver function and liver histology, and alleviation of symptoms associated with primary biliary cirrhosis[4].

Bile acid synthesis from cholesterol can occur via two pathways (Fig. 1). The *neutral* bile acid biosynthetic pathway has been considered, until recently, to be the main pathway for bile acid synthesis. It involves 14 enzymatic reactions taking place in four different organelles, a process in which water-insoluble molecules of cholesterol are converted to water-soluble molecules of cholic or chenodeoxycholic acids. The initial and rate-determining step in the neutral bile acid biosynthetic pathway is conversion of cholesterol to 7α-hydroxycholesterol. This reaction is catalysed by cholesterol 7α-hydroxylase, a microsomal P450 monooxygenase, an enzyme found exclusively in the liver. This enzyme has recently been characterized, cloned and sequenced[5-7]. Subsequent studies have demonstrated that cholesterol 7α-hydroxylase is regulated by several effector molecules, such as hydrophobic bile acids[8-13], cholesterol[14,15], glucocorticoids, thyroxine and glucagon[16], all at the level of gene transcription.

CHOLESTEROL DEGRADATION TO BILE ACIDS AND MAIN ENZYMES INVOLVED IN BILE ACID BIOSYNTHESIS

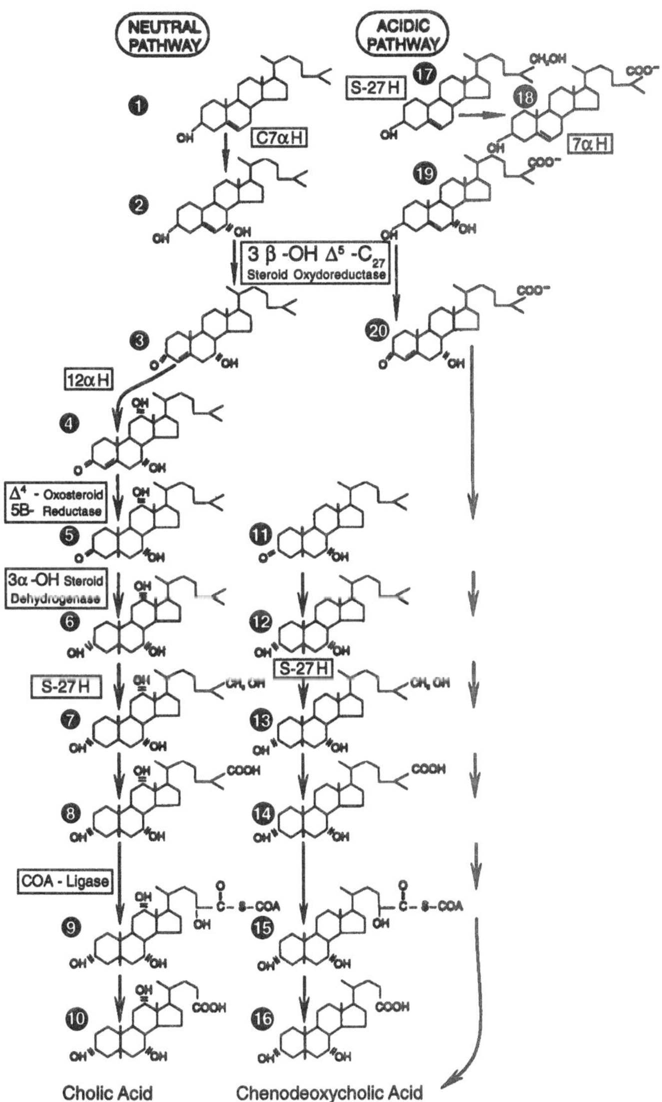

Fig. 1 Neutral and acidic pathways of bile (C7αH) catalyse the initial step in the neutral pathway, i.e. conversion of cholesterol to 7α-hydroxycholesterol (step 1). Mitochondrial sterol 27-hydroxylase (S-27H) catalyses the initial step in the acidic pathway, i.e. conversion of cholesterol to 27-hydroxycholesterol (step 17). 27-H also initiates side-chain oxidation bile acid intermediates (5β-cholestane 3α,7α,12α-triol and 5β-cholestane 3α,7α-diol) in the neutral pathway (step 6 and 12, respectively). The intermediates of the acidic pathway in which side-chain oxidation has been initiated undergo hydroxylation at C-7 position by a microsomal or mitochondrial 7α-hydroxylase (7αH) which is different from cholesterol 7α-hydroxylase (step 18)

It has been known for some time that bile acids returning to the liver, via portal circulation, regulate cholesterol 7α-hydroxylase and hence their own synthesis via the negative feedback control[17–19]. Complete or partial biliary diversion causes a diminished return of bile acids to the liver, resulting in up-regulation of cholesterol 7α-hydroxylase-specific activity and an increase in bile acid synthesis. In contrast, hydrophobic bile acid, administered orally, results in an increase of return of bile acids to the liver, down-regulation of cholesterol 7α-hydroxylase specific activity and reduced endogenous synthesis of bile acids[20]. Recent studies have shown that only hydrophobic bile acids down-regulate cholesterol 7α-hydroxylase, while hydrophilic bile acids have no effect [9,10]. Pandak *et al.*[11,12] and Stravitz *et al.*[13] demonstrated that bile acids regulate cholesterol 7α-hydroxylase predominantly at the level of gene transcription. The exact interaction of bile acids with the $5'$-flanking region of cholesterol 7α-hydroxylase gene has not been fully studied. Bile acids could interact with the $5'$-flanking region *directly*, i.e. by binding to cytosolic bile acid receptors, which enter the nucleus and interact with bile acid responsive element (BARE)[21,22]. This explanation is not likely, since there is no evidence that bile acids bound to the receptors enter the nucleus. Alternatively, bile acids could activate the second messenger system which phosphorylates a transcription factor which then interacts with the $5'$-flanking region of cholesterol 7α-hydroxylase gene (indirect effect). Recent data from Stravitz *et al.*[23] provide evidence which suggests that cholesterol 7α-hydroxylase is regulated by hydrophobic bile acids via activation of several isoforms of protein kinase C. These studies suggest that activation of protein kinase C is triggered by hydrophobic, but not hydrophilic, bile acids, and provide a plausible explanation for the previously observed role of bile acid hydrophobicity in the regulation of cholesterol 7α-hydroxylase.

Studies in primary rat hepatocytes have shown convincingly that addition of physiological concentrations of dexamethasone and thyroxine increase cholesterol 7α-hydroxylase-specific activity, mRNA level and gene transcriptional activity several-fold[16]. The addition of dexamethasone and thyroxine alone does not alter significantly any of the above parameters. The reason for the synergistic action of these two hormones which results in the stimulation of cholesterol 7α-hydroxylase gene transcription has not been clarified. These *in vitro* data have been confirmed by *in vivo* data in which we have shown that hypophysectomy, or thyroidectomy plus hypophysectomy, resulted in a decrease of cholesterol 7α-hydroxylase-specific activity, steady-state mRNA levels and gene transcriptional activity. In contrast, thyroidectomy or adrenalectomy alone failed to significantly alter any of these three parameters[24]. The addition of physiological concentrations of glucagon suppressed cholesterol 7α-hydroxylase mRNA level and gene transcriptional activity in primary rat hepatocytes. The suppression is concentration-dependent and can be reproduced by the addition of cyclic AMP. These data suggest that glucagon also affects cholesterol 7α-hydroxylase by activation of the second messenger system[16]. Infusion of varying concentrations of glucagon to rats with chronic bile fistula resulted in a concentration-dependent decrease in cholesterol 7α-hydroxylase-specific activity, mRNA and gene transcriptional activity, as well as bile acid synthesis. In contrast, enteroglucagon had no effect on cholesterol 7α-hydroxylase-specific activity or bile acid synthesis (unpublished observations). Thus *in vivo* and *in vitro* data suggest that glucagon may be another physiological regulator of cholesterol 7α-hydroxylase.

Feeding of 2% cholesterol in the diet results in a marked increase of cholesterol 7α-hydroxylase-specific activity, mRNA levels and gene transcriptional activity[11,14]. Because of reports that cholesterol feeding could cause bile acid malabsorption[25], we carried out studies in which intestinal effects of cholesterol feeding were circumvented by intravenous infusion of mevalonate, a precursor of cholesterol, to rats with intact enterohepatic circulation for 3, 6, 12, and 24 h. The results of this study suggest that at all time periods mevalonate, an intermediate in the cholesterol biosynthetic pathway which is rapidly converted to cholesterol, increases cholesterol 7α-hydroxylase-specific activity, mRNA levels and gene transcription. Conversely, the inhibition of cholesterol synthesis with lovastatin in rats with chronic bile fistula and high rates of cholesterol synthesis resulted in marked decrease in cholesterol 7α-hydroxylase-specific activity, enzyme mass, steady-state mRNA levels and gene transcriptional activity in rats[14]. Addition of squalestatin to primary rat hepatocytes caused a concentration-dependent decrease of cholesterol 7α-hydroxylase mRNA levels. At higher concentrations of squalestatin cholesterol 7α-hydroxylase mRNA was barely detectable; the addition of increasing concentrations of cholesterol to these primary rat hepatocytes with repressed cholesterol 7α-hydroxylase mRNA levels resulted in return of these levels to normal (unpublished observations). These *in vivo* and *in vitro* data provide strong evidence that, at least in the rat, under the circumstances in which cholesterol is present in excess, cholesterol 7α-hydroxylase is up-regulated and degradation of cholesterol to bile acids is facilitated. Conversely, when cholesterol availability is decreased, cholesterol 7α-hydroxylase is suppressed, leading to a decrease in cholesterol elimination. This finely tuned mechanism provides a plausible explanation about the regulation of cholesterol homeostasis in the rat. However, the effects of cholesterol on cholesterol 7α-hydroxylase appears to be species-specific. In the hamster, feeding a diet high in cholesterol resulted in repression, rather than stimulation, of cholesterol 7α-hydroxylase-specific activity, mRNA and gene transcriptional activity (unpublished observation). These findings provide a plausible explanation for the observation that a diet high in cholesterol does not cause hypercholesterolaemia in the rat, but is associated with a marked increase in serum cholesterol in the hamster. In light of the propensity of humans to develop hypercholesterolaemia as a result of high cholesterol intake, hepatic cholesterol metabolism in this species may be more akin to hamsters than to rats.

Cholesterol degradation to bile acids via the so-called *acidic* pathway results in predominant synthesis of chenodeoxycholic acid. The first step in this pathway is conversion of cholesterol to 27-hydroxycholesterol. This reaction is catalysed by mitochondrial sterol 27-hydroxylase, a P450 enzyme which also participates in the initiation of side-chain oxidation of bile acid intermediates in the neutral pathway[26]. Contrary to cholesterol 7α-hydroxylase, sterol 27-hydroxylase is ubiquitous, as it has been found in tissues other than the liver such as duodenum, kidney, fibrocytes, etc[27,28]. 27-Hydroxycholesterol, a product of hydroxylation of cholesterol at C-27, is an oxysterol which circulates in the plasma incorporated into low-density lipoproteins[29]. 27-Hydroxylase is a powerful inhibitor of low-density lipoprotein, HMG-CoA reductase and HMG-CoA-synthase transcription[30–32]. Mitochondrial sterol 27-hydroxylase has recently been purified and cloned[27,28]. This enzyme is deficient or absent in cerebrotendinous xanthomatosis, an inborn error of bile acid synthesis, a disease with low rates of bile acid synthesis[33]. Bile acid synthesis via acidic pathway was thought to be insignificant in adults until Axelson and co-workers[34–36] recently demonstrated the presence of circulating levels of the intermediates of the acidic pathway in plasma of human subjects. These investigators postulated that, under normal circumstances, the neutral pathway is a major contributor to bile acid synthesis. However, in conditions in which bile acid synthesis is low, such as in cirrhosis of the liver or cholestatis, the contribution of acidic pathway to total bile acid synthesis may be of greater magnitude. Feeding cholestyramine to humans resulted in a marked increase in the intermediates of the neutral, but not the acidic, pathway in plasma, leading the authors to postulate that sterol 27-hydroxylase is probably not regulated by the negative feedback control[36]. Princen *et al.*[37,38] have shown that cyclosporin, a specific inhibitor of conversion of cholesterol to 27-hydroxycholesterol (but not of 27-hydroxylation of bile acid intermediates in the neutral pathway) results in a 50% decrease of bile acid synthesis in primary rat and human hepatocytes. These authors interpreted these findings as evidence that, in the primary rat or human hepatocytes, the acidic pathway contributes approximately 50% of bile acids to total bile acid synthesis. These results are in agreement with our own data in primary rat hepatocytes using different experimental techniques (not published).

We have recently completed a series of *in vivo* studies on the regulation of sterol 27-hydroxylase by bile acids and compared the data to those obtained with cholesterol 7α-hydroxylase (unpublished observation). Partial biliary diversion after use of cholestyramine increased sterol 27-hydroxylase-specific activity, mRNA and gene transcriptional activity significantly, albeit the changes were not nearly as marked as those observed with cholesterol 7α-hydroxylase. Similarly, 14 days of feeding of cholic, chenodeoxycholic and deoxycholic acids (ranging between 0.25% and 1%) resulted in marked repression of sterol 27-hydroxylase-specific activity, mRNA levels and gene transcription. The extent of repression of sterol 27-hydroxylase was less prominent than that of cholesterol 7α-hydroxylase. Both cholesterol 7α-hydroxylase and sterol 27-hydroxylase undergo diurnal variation, suggesting that glucocorticoids also play a role in the regulation of both enzymes. The effects of glucocorticoids, thyroxine, glucagon and cholesterol on sterol 27-hydroxylase are not known. Similarly, we have observed that complete biliary diversion (days 3 and 5) leads to marked increases of sterol 27-hydroxylase-specific activity and mRNA levels, which again were not as pronounced as those of cholesterol 7α-hydroxylase.

In summary, in the last 4–5 years we have learned a great deal about the regulation of bile acid synthesis. It appears that cholesterol can be converted to bile acids via the neutral pathway with the main end-products of cholic and chenodeoxycholic acids, or via the acidic pathway with the main end-product of chenodeoxycholic acid. It is not clear what the contribution of each pathway is to total bile acid synthesis, or whether the synthesis of bile acid via both pathways is altered in diseases of the liver. The data obtained so far provide strong evidence that both cholesterol 7α-hydroxylase and sterol 27-hydroxylase are

Regulation of Cholesterol 7α-Hydroxylase (C7αH)
1994

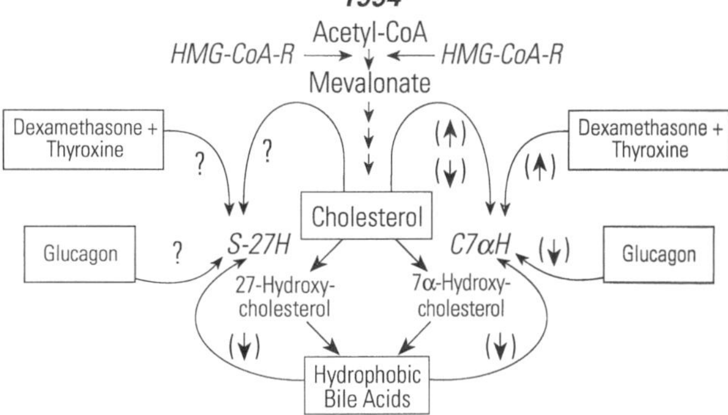

Fig. 2 Schematic presentation of regulation of cholesterol 7α-hydroxylase and sterol 27-hydroxylase (S-27H). C7αH and S-27H are both regulated by bile acids via negative feedback control. C7αH is also regulated by cholestane, thyroid and glucocorticoids and glucagon. The extent of regulation of S-27H by these latter effectors is not known

subject to negative bile acid biofeedback control by hydrophobic bile acids, and are probably regulated by glucocorticoids (Fig. 2). Determination of the molecular basis of regulation of sterol 27-hydroxylase by different effectors will be the next target of scientific investigation.

References

1. Vlahcevic ZR, Heuman DM, Hylemon PB. Physiology and pathophysiology of enterohepatic circulation of bile acids. In: Zakim D, Boyer T, editors. Hepatology: a textbook of liver disease, 2nd edn, vol 1. Philadelphia: Saunders; 1990:341–77.
2. Heuman DM, Pandak WM, Hylemon PB, Vlahcevic ZR. Conjugates of ursodeoxycholate protect against cytotoxicity of more hydrophobic bile salts: *in vitro* studies in rat hepatocytes and human erythrocytes. Hepatology. 1991;14:920–6.
3. Heuman DM. Editorial: Hepatoprotective properties of ursodeoxycholate. Gastroenterology. 1993;104:1865–70.
4. Poupon RE, Balkav B, Eschwège E, Poupon R. UDCA–PBC Study Group. A multicenter controlled trial of ursodiol for the treatment of primary biliary cirrhosis. N Engl J Med. 1991;324:1548–54.
5. Noshiro M, Nishimoto M, Morohashi K, Okuda K. Molecular cloning of cDNA for cholesterol 7α-hydroxylase from microsomes. FEBS Lett. 1989;257:97–100.
6. Li YC, Wang DP, Chiang JYL. Regulation of cholesterol 7α-hydroxylase in the liver: cloning, sequencing and regulation of cholesterol 7α-hydroxylase mRNA. J Biol Chem. 1990;265:12012–19.
7. Jelinek DF, Russell DW. Structure of the rat gene encoding cholesterol 7α-hydroxylase. Biochemistry. 1990;29:7781–5.
8. Heuman DM, Hernandez, CR, Hylemon PB, Kubaska W, Hartmann C, Vlahcevic ZR. Regulation of bile acid synthesis. I. Effects of conjugated ursodeoxycholate and cholate on bile acid synthesis in chronic bile fistula rat. Hepatology. 1988;8:358–65.
9. Heuman DM, Vlahcevic ZR, Bailey ML, Hylemon PB. Regulation of bile acid synthesis. II. Effect of bile acid feeding on enzymes regulating hepatic cholesterol and bile acid synthesis in the rat. Hepatology. 1988;8:892–7.
10. Heuman DM, Hylemon PB, Vlahcevic ZR. Regulation of bile acid synthesis. III. Correlation between biliary bile salt hydrophobicity index and the activities of enzymes regulating cholesterol and bile acid synthesis in the rat. J Lipid Res. 1989;30:1161–71.

11. Pandak WM, Li YC, Chiang JYL *et al*. Regulation of cholesterol 7α-hydroxylase mRNA and transcriptional activity by taurocholate and cholesterol in the chronic biliary diverted rat. J Biol Chem. 1991;266:3416–21.

12. Pandak WM, Vlahcevic ZR, Heuman DM, Redford KS, Chiang JYL, Hylemon PB. Effects of different bile salts on the steady state mRNA levels and transcriptional activity of cholesterol 7α-hydroxylase. Hepatology. 1994;19:941–7.

13. Stravitz R, Hylemon PB, Heuman DM *et al*. Transcriptional regulation of cholesterol 7α-hydroxylase mRNA by conjugated bile acids in primary cultures of rat hepatocytes. J Biol Chem. 1993;268:13987–93.

14. Jones MP, Pandak WM, Heuman DM, Chiang JYL, Hylemon PB, Vlahcevic ZR. Cholesterol 7α-hydroxylase: evidence for transcriptional regulation by cholesterol in the rat. J Lipid Res. 1993;34:885–92.

15. Vlahcevic ZR, Pandak WM, Hylemon PB, Heuman DM. Role of newly synthesized cholesterol or its metabolites on the regulation of bile acid biosynthesis following acute biliary diversion in the rat. Hepatology. 1993;18:660–8.

16. Hylemon PB, Gurley EC, Stravitz RT *et al*. Hormonal regulation of cholesterol 7α-hydroxylase mRNA levels and transcriptional activity in primary rat hepatocyte cultures. J Biol Chem. 1992;267:16866–71.

17. Danielsson H, Einarsson K, Johansson G. Effect of biliary drainage on individual reactions in the conversion of cholesterol to taurocholic acid. Bile acids and steroids 180. Eur J Biochem. 1967;2:44–9.

18. Shefer S, Hauser S, Bekersky I, Mosbach EH. Feedback regulation of bile acid biosynthesis on the rat. J Lipid Res. 1969;10:646–55.

19. Shefer S, Hauser S, Lapar V, Mosbach EH. Regulatory effects of sterols and bile acids on hepatic 3-hydroxy-3-methylglutaryl CoA reductase and cholesterol 7α-hydroxylase in the rat. J Lipid Res. 1973;14:573–80.

20. Russell DW, Setchell KDR. Bile acid biosynthesis. Biochemistry. 1992;31:4737–49.

21. Molowa DT, Chen WS, Cimis GM, Tan CP. Transcriptional regulation of the human cholesterol 7α-hydroxylase gene. Biochemistry. 1992;31:2539–44.

22. Hoekman MFM, Rientjes JMJ, Twisk J, Planta RJ, Princen HMG, Mager WH. Transcriptional regulation of the gene encoding cholesterol 7α-hydroxylase in the rat. Gene. 1993;130:217–23.

23. Stravitz RT, Vlahcevic ZR, Gurley EC, Hylemon PB. Repression of cholesterol 7α-hydroxylase transcription by bile acids is mediated through protein kinase C in primary rat hepatocytes. J Lipid Res (Submitted).

24. Vlahcevic ZR, Stravitz RT, Gurley EC, Pandak WM, Hylemon PB. *In vitro* and *in vivo* studies of hormonal regulation of cholesterol 7α-hydroxylase. In: Paumgartner G, Stiehl A, Gerok W, editors. Bile acids and the hepatobiliary system. Falk Symposium 68. Dordrecht: Kluwer; 1993:33–43.

25. Björkem I, Eggertsen G, Andersson U. On the mechanism of stimulation of cholesterol 7α-hydroxylase by dietary cholesterol. Biochem Biophys Acta. 1991;1085:329–35.

26. Björkem I. Mechanism of degradation of steroid side chain in formation of bile acids. J Lipid Res. 1992;33:455–71.

27. Andersson S, Davis DL, Dahlback H, Jörnvall H, Russell DW. Cloning, structure, and expression of the mitochondrial cytochrome P-450 sterol 26-hydroxylase, a bile acid biosynthetic enzyme. J Biol Chem. 1989;264:8222–9.

28. Cali JJ, Russell DW. Characterization of human sterol 27-hydroxylase. J Biol Chem. 1991;266:7774–8.

29. Javitt NB, Kok E, Burstein S, Cohen B, Kutscher J. 26-hydroxycholesterol. Identification and quantitation in human serum. J Biol Chem. 1981;56:12644–6.

30. Osborne TF, Goldstein JL, Brown MS. 5′ end of HMG CoA reductase gene contains sequences responsible for cholesterol inhibition of transcription. Cell. 1985;42:203–12.

31. Smith JR, Osborne TF, Brown MS, Goldstein JL, Gil G. Multiple sterol regulatory elements in promoter for hamster 3-hydroxy-3-methylglutaryl-coenzyme A synthase. J Biol Chem. 1988;263:18480–7.

32. Südhof TC, Russell DW, Brown MS, Goldstein JL. 42 bp element from LDL receptor gene confers end-product repression by sterols when inserted into viral TK promoter. Cell. 1987;48:1061–9.

33. Cali JJ, Hsieh C-L, Francke U, Russell DW. Mutations in the bile acid biosynthetic enzyme sterol 27-hydroxylase underlie cerebrotendinous xanthomatosis. J Biol Chem. 1991;266:7779–83.
34. Axelson M, Sjövall J. Potential bile acid precursors in plasma – possible indicators of biosynthetic pathways to cholic and chenodeoxycholic acids in man. J Steroid Biochem. 1990;36:631–40.
35. Axelson M, Mörk B, Sjövall J. Studies on biosynthetic pathway to cholic and chenodeoxycholic acids in humans. In: Bile acids as therapeutic agents. Falk Symposium 58. Norwell (MA) Kluwer; 1991:53–62.
36. Axelson M, Mörk B, Sjövall J. Occurrence of 3ß-hydroxy-5-cholestenoic acid, 3ß,7α-dihydroxy-5-cholestenoic acid and 7α-hydroxy-oxo-4-cholestenoic acid as normal constituents on human blood. J Lipid Res. 1988;29:629–41.
37. Princen HMG, Meijer P, Wolthers BG, Vonk RJ, Kuipers F. Cyclosporin A blocks bile acid synthesis in cultured hepatocytes by inhibition of chenodeoxycholic acid and ß muricholic acid synthesis. Biochem J. 1991;275:501–5.
38. Dahlbäck-Sjöberg H, Björkem I, Princen HMG. Selective inhibition of mitochondrial 27-hydroxylation of bile acid intermediates and 25-hydroxylation of vitamin D3 by cyclosporine A. Biochem J. 1993;293:203–6.

Section II
Bile acid transport

4
Hepatocellular basolateral bile acid uptake proteins

B. HAGENBUCH, B. STIEGER and P. J. MEIER

INTRODUCTION

An important function of the liver is the excretion of potentially toxic amphipathic organic anions into bile. Quantitatively the bile acids represent the major cholephilic organic compounds. Their basolateral uptake into hepatocytes is mediated by Na^+-dependent as well as Na^+-independent transport pathways[1]. Functionally these hepatocellular bile acid uptake systems have been well characterized in a number of experimental systems including the perfused rat liver[2], isolated and cultured hepatocytes[3,4], and basolateral liver plasma membrane vesicles[5-7]. In addition, identification and isolation of the involved bile acid transporting polypeptides have been attempted by photoaffinity labelling and immunochemical studies[8-14]. These studies first suggested proteins in the molecular weight range of 48–54 kDa as essential components of the basolateral bile acid uptake systems[8-10]. However, classical biochemical techniques based on solubilization and functional reconstitution into proteoliposomes proved to be unsuitable for the unequivocal successful identification and isolation of the hepatocellular Na^+-dependent and Na^+-independent bile acid and/or bromosulphophthalein (BSP) uptake systems. Therefore we used the strategy of expression cloning in *Xenopus laevis* oocytes to isolate a Na^+-dependent bile acid uptake[15,16] and a Na^+-independent bile acid uptake system[17,18] from rat and human liver.

Na⁺/TAUROCHOLATE COTRANSPORTING POLYPEPTIDE (Ntcp/NTCP)

The cloned hepatocellular Na^+-bile acid cotransporter consists of 362 amino acids with five consensus sites for N-linked glycosylation (Fig. 1)[15]. Recent experiments using site-directed mutagenesis revealed that only asparagins at positions 5 and 11 are glycosylated. As a consequence the amino terminal end of Ntcp is most probably located on the extracellular side of the plasma mem-

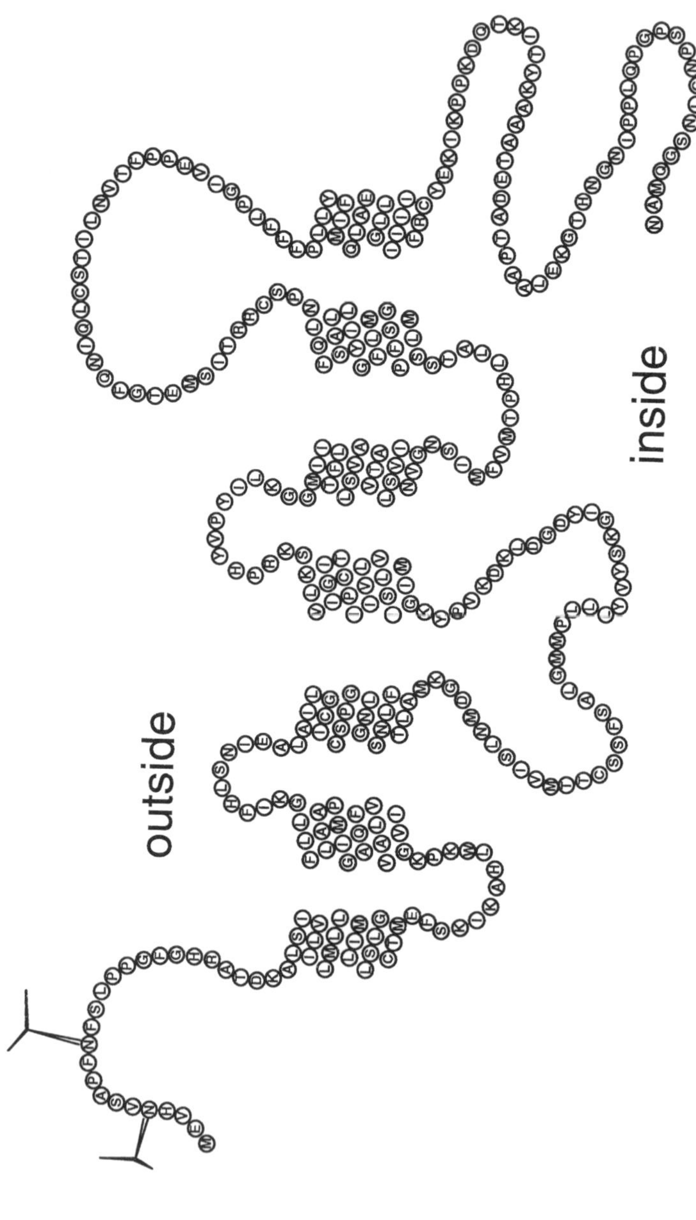

Fig. 1 Model of the rat hepatic Ntcp. The primary amino acid sequence of Ntcp is arranged in a secondary structure model. The N-terminal end is on the extracellular side and the C-terminal end on the cytoplasmic side of the membrane. The two N-glycosylation sites (see text) are indicated

brane. A polyclonal antibody against a fusion protein containing the maltose-binding protein of *E. coli* and 56 amino acids of the C-terminal end of Ntcp yielded a positive immunoreaction only in detergent-permeabilized rat hepatocytes[19]. This finding indicates that the C-terminal end of Ntcp is located on the cytoplasmic side of the membrane. Thus, although hydrophobicity analysis alone yields six, seven or eight transmembrane domains, depending on the algorithm used[20–22], only the seven transmembrane topology of Ntcp is consistent with an extra- and intracellular localization of the N- and C-terminal ends, respectively. Therefore, we conclude that the rat Ntcp (and the human NTCP) is a seven transmembrane domain glycoprotein (Fig. 1) with structural similarities to the protein superfamilies of rhodopsin[23] and the G protein-linked receptors[24], which also have seven transmembrane domains, but no significant sequence homology to Ntcp. *In-vitro* translation experiments revealed an apparent molecular weight of 33 kDa for the unglycosylated and 39 kDa for the glycosylated Ntcp[15]. However, since *in-vitro* translation cannot account for complex glycosylation, the molecular weight of the native protein was immunologically determined in isolated rat liver basolateral membranes with an Ntcp-specific polyclonal antibody. In Western blots, native Ntcp showed an apparent molecular weight of 51 kDa which, after deglycosylation of isolated basolateral membranes, decreased to 33.5 kDa[19]. The latter value is similar to the molecular weight previously obtained after *in-vitro* translation of Ntcp-cRNA in the absence of dog pancreatic microsomes[15]. Using the same antibody, it has also been shown that Ntcp is selectively localized to the basolateral plasma membrane of rat hepatocytes[19].

In order to more definitely characterize its transport properties Ntcp was transiently or stably expressed in several eukaryotic cell lines, including COS-7[25], MDCK, CHO and V79 cells[26]. These studies demonstrated very consistent K_m values for Ntcp-mediated Na^+-dependent taurocholate transport between 25 and 42 μmol/l. In addition, Ntcp can also transport some non-bile acid organic anions such as oestrone-3-sulphate[27]. However, these studies failed to demonstrate transport of bumetanide and cyclosporin A by Ntcp, although both these substrates have been reported to competitively inhibit Na^+-dependent taurocholate uptake into isolated hepatocytes and in liver plasma membrane vesicles[28,29]. Hence, although Ntcp appears to possess a broad substrate specificity, the spectrum of transported substrates is nevertheless limited, and can obviously not be adequately derived from kinetic *cis*-inhibition studies alone.

Based on Northern blot analysis, Ntcp is present only in mammalian liver[30]. It is not expressed in the liver of lower vertebrates, which is also devoid of functional Na^+-dependent taurocholate uptake. This late phylogenic expression of Ntcp is mirrored by a similar late ontogenic expression in developing rat liver[30]. In adult liver, Ntcp expression is down-regulated during cholestasis, liver regeneration and pregnancy[31–34]. A marked increase of Ntcp expression, however, is seen post partum and during prolactin treatment of ovariectomized rats[35]. Prolactin is the only endogenous up-regulator of Ntcp expression so far identified. The tissue distribution of Ntcp was also evaluated by Northern blot experiments. Positive reactivity with renal mRNA[15] indicated that a similar bile acid transport system may also occur in the kidney.

The human NTCP, which was isolated by hybridization screening of a human liver cDNA library with the rat probe, exhibits 77% amino acid identity to the rat protein[16]. Like the rat system the human NTCP transports all major bile acids tested in a Na^+-dependent manner. However, its affinity for taurocholate is about 4–6-fold higher ($K_m = 6$ μmol/l) than that of the rat transport system. The gene coding for NTCP is located on chromosome 14.

ORGANIC ANION TRANSPORTING POLYPEPTIDE (oatp/OATP)

Using the same cloning strategy a Na^+-independent BSP and bile acid uptake system could also be isolated from rat liver[17]. The protein consists of 670 amino acids with four potential N-linked glycosylation sites and 10–12 transmembrane domains[20–22]. Since many transport proteins are predicted to have 12 transmembrane domains[36] we are using the topology shown in Fig. 2 as a working model. Antipeptide antibodies recognized an 80 kDa protein on Western blots of sinusoidal but not canalicular rat liver plasma membranes[37]. On liver sections, immunostaining was restricted to the basolateral plasma membrane[37]. Functionally, oatp is a transport protein with a broad substrate specificity. Besides BSP and bile acids[17,38] oatp also mediates Na^+-independent transport of oestrogen conjugates and ouabain (Bossuyet *et al.* in preparation). Northern blot analysis of different rat tissues revealed several transcripts in liver and kidney, as well as hybridization with brain, lung, skeletal muscle and proximal colon[17]. These multiple transcripts in liver and kidney indicate that there are additional, oatp-related proteins which might transport other, or additional, so far unidentified organic anions.

The human OATP, which was isolated by hybridization screening of a human liver cDNA library, exhibits 67% amino acid identity to the rat protein[18]. Functionally, it also mediates Na^+-independent BSP and bile acid uptake. It is also inhibited by all the substrates that inhibit the rat protein with the exception of bilirubin and probenecid. On Northern blots OATP cDNA hybridized with mRNA of brain, kidney, liver, lung and testis. The gene for OATP has been localized to chromosome 12.

CONCLUSIONS

Our studies demonstrated that expression cloning in *Xenopus laevis* oocytes is a very effective approach for the cloning of hepatocytic basolateral membrane transport systems. The cloned Na^+-dependent bile acid uptake system is an exclusive function of differentiated mammalian hepatocytes. Its expression appears to be regulated and, at least in part, under hormonal control (e.g. prolactin stimulation). In addition, the substrate specificity of Ntcp appears to be restricted, although Ntcp can mediate transport of some non-bile acid organic anions. Although preliminary studies with antisense oligonucleotides suggest that Ntcp represents the major Na^+-dependent bile acid uptake system of rat liver, the coexistence of additional hepatic Na^+-dependent bile acid transporters cannot yet be excluded. In addition, it remains to be seen whether Ntcp-mediated bile acid transport has any direct effects on the degree of differen-

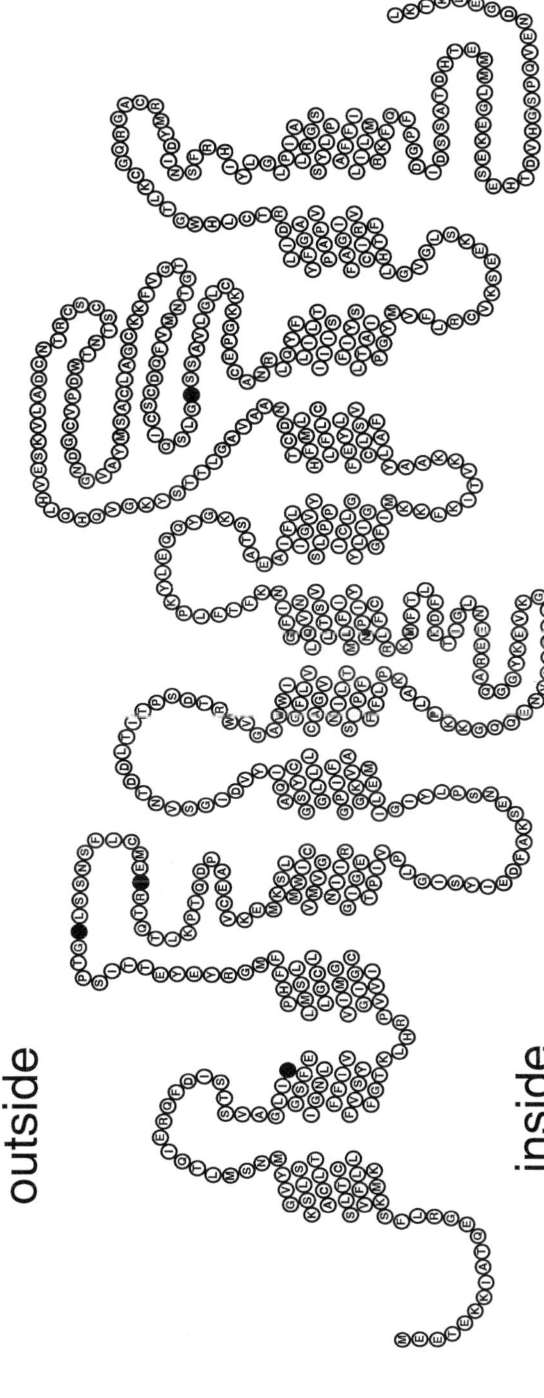

Fig. 2 Model of the rat hepatic oatp. The primary amino acid sequence of oatp is shown arranged in a secondary structure model with 12 transmembrane domains. The amino terminal end is in the cytoplasm and the four potential N-linked glycosylation sites are marked by the filled circles

tiation of hepatocytes *per se*; oatp demonstrates a strikingly broader spectrum of transported substrates and a considerable wider tissue distribution than Ntcp. These features indicate a major fundamental role of oatp in transepithelial organic substrate transport of various organs. Furthermore, in Northern blots several reactive mRNA species were detected, indicating that there are additional 'oatp-related' transporting polypeptides present in various organs. However, these hypothetical transporters remain to be identified and cloned. In addition, further experiments are required to investigate the phylogenic and ontogenic development of oatp, as well as to define more clearly the putative transport role of oatp in extrahepatic tissues.

Acknowledgements

This study was supported by the Swiss National Science Foundation Grant 32-29878.90 (to P.J.M.). Dr B. Hagenbuch is a recipient of a Cloetta Foundation Fellowship.

References

1. Suchy FJ. Hepatocellular transport of bile acids. Semin Liver Dis. 1993;13:235–47.
2. Reichen J, Paumgartner G. Uptake of bile acids by perfused rat liver. Am J Physiol. 1976;231:734–42.
3. Schwarz LR, Burr R, Schwenk M, Pfaff E, Greim H. Uptake of taurocholic acid into isolated rat liver cells. Eur J Biochem. 1975;55:617–23.
4. Van Dyke RW, Stephens JE, Scharschmidt BF. Bile acid transport in cultured rat hepatocytes. Am J Physiol. 1982;243:G484–92.
5. Inoue M, Kinne R, Tran T, Arias IM. Taurocholate transport by rat liver sinusoidal membrane vesicles: evidence for sodium cotransport. Hepatology. 1982;2:572–9.
6. Zimmerli B, Valantinas J, Meier PJ. Multispecificity of Na$^+$-dependent taurocholate uptake in basolateral (sinusoidal) rat liver plasma membrane vesicles. J Pharmacol Exp Ther. 1989; 250:301–8.
7. Novak DA, Ryckman FC, Suchy FJ. Taurocholate transport by basolateral plasma membrane vesicles isolated from human liver. Hepatology. 1989;10:447–53.
8. Kramer W, Bickel U, Buscher H-P, Gerok W, Kurz G. Bile-salt-binding polypeptides in plasma membranes of hepatocytes revealed by photoaffinity labelling. Eur J Biochem. 1982;129:13–24.
9. Wieland T, Nassal M, Kramer W, Fricker G, Bickel U, Kurz G. Identity of hepatic membrane transport systems for bile salts, phalloidin, and antamanide by photoaffinity labeling. Proc Natl Acad Sci USA. 1984;81:5232–6.
10. von Dippe P, Levy D. Characterization of the bile acid transport system in normal and transformed hepatocytes. J Biol Chem. 1983;258:8896–901.
11. Ananthanarayanan M, von Dippe P, Levy D. Identification of the hepatocyte Na$^+$-dependent bile acid transport protein using monoclonal antibodies. J Biol Chem. 1988;263;8338–43.
12. von Dippe P, Levy D. Reconstitution of the immunopurified 49-kDa sodium-dependent bile acid transport protein derived from hepatocytes sinusoidal plasma membranes. J Biol Chem. 1990;265;14812–16.
13. Ananthanarayanan M, Bucuvalas JC, Shneider BL, Sippel CJ, Suchy FJ. An ontogenically regulated 48-kDa protein is a component of the Na$^+$-bile acid cotransporter of rat liver. Am J Physiol. 1991;261:G810–17.
14. Berk PD, Potter BJ, Stremmel W. Role of plasma membrane ligand-binding proteins in the hepatocellular uptake of albumin-bound organic anions. Hepatology. 1987;7:165–76.
15. Hagenbuch B, Stieger B, Foguet M, Lübbert H, Meier PJ. Functional expression cloning and characterization of the hepatocyte Na$^+$/bile acid cotransport system. Proc Natl Acad Sci USA. 1991;88:10629–33.
16. Hagenbuch B, Meier PJ. Molecular cloning, chromosomal localization, and functional characterization of a human liver Na$^+$ bile acid contransporter. J Clin Invest. 1994;93:1326–31.

17. Jacquemin E, Hagenbuch B, Stieger B, Wolkoff AW, Meier PJ. Expression cloning of a rat liver Na$^+$-independent organic anion transporter. Proc Natl Acad Sci USA. 1994;91:133–7.
18. Kullak-Ublick GA, Hagenbuch B, Stieger B *et al*. Molecular and functional characterization of an organic anion transporting polypeptide cloned from human liver. (Submitted.)
19. Stieger B, Hagenbuch B, Landmann L, Höchli M, Schroeder A, Meier PJ. *In situ* localization of the hepatocytic Na$^+$/taurocholate cotransporting polypeptide (Ntcp) in rat liver. Gastroenterology. 1994;107:1781–7.
20. Kyte J, Doolittle RF. A simple method for displaying the hydropathic character of a protein. J Mol Biol. 1982;157:105–32.
21. Klein P, Kanehisa M, DeLisi C. The detection and classification of membrane-spanning proteins. Biochim Biophys Acta. 1985;815:468–76.
22. Eisenberg D, Schwarz E, Komaromy M, Wall R. Analysis of membrane and surface protein sequences with the hydrophobic moment plot. J Mol Biol. 1984;179:125–42.
23. Khorana HG. Rhodopsin, photoreceptor of the rod cell. J Biol Chem. 1992;267:1–4.
24. Findlay J, Eliopoulos E. Three-dimensional modelling of G protein-linked receptors. TiPS. 1990;11:492–9.
25. Boyer JL, Ng OC, Ananthanarayanan M *et al*. Expression and characterization of a functional rat liver Na$^+$ bile acid cotransport system in COS-7 cells. Am J Physiol. 1994;266:G382–7.
26. Stieger B, Hagenbuch B, Cornacchia L, Schroeder A, Landmann L, Meier PJ. Molecular properties of the Na$^+$-dependent taurocholate cotransporting polypeptide (Ntcp) of rat liver. Hepatology. 1993;18:S6.
27. Schroeder A, Hagenbuch B, Stieger B *et al*. The rat hepatocyte Na$^+$/taurocholate cotransporting polypeptide (Ntcp) mediates multispecific substrate transport in stably transfected chinese hamster ovary (CHO) cells. Gastroenterology. 1994;106;A979.
28. Petzinger E, Mueller N, Foellmann W, Deutscher J, Kinne RKH. Uptake of bumetanide into isolated rat hepatocytes and primary liver cell cultures. Am J Physiol. 1989;256:G78–86.
29. Moseley RH, Johnson TR, Morrissette JM. Inhibition of bile acid transport by cyclosporine A in rat liver plasma membrane vesicles. J Pharmacol Exp Ther. 1990;253:974–80.
30. Boyer JL, Hagenbuch B, Ananthanarayanan M, Suchy F, Stieger B, Meier PJ. Phylogenic and ontogenic expression of hepatocellular bile acid transport. Proc Natl Acad Sci USA. 1993;90:435–8.
31. Gartung C, Ananthanarayanan M, Rahman MA, Stolz A, Suchy FJ, Boyer JL. Cholestasis induces downregulation of the sodium-dependent bile acid (BA) cotransporter and cytosolic binding proteins following bile duct ligation (BDL) in the rat. Hepatology. 1993;18:139A.
32. Kupferschmidt H, Hagenbuch B, Stieger B, Kraehenbühl S, Meier PJ. Ethinylestradiol induces differential effects on various transporter mRNA and protein levels in rat liver. Hepatology. 1994;20:175A.
33. Green RM, Lipin Al, Pelletier EM *et al*. Hepatic regeneration is associated with a marked reduction in mRNA expression of the basolateral Na$^+$-taurocholate transporter. Gastroenterology. 1994;106:A901.
34. Ganguly T, Hyde JF, Vore M. Prolactin increases Na$^+$/taurocholate cotransport in isolated hepatocytes from postpartum rats and ovariectomized rats. J Pharmacol Exp Ther. 1993;267:82–7.
35. Ganguly TC, Liu Y, Hyde JF, Hagenbuch B, Meier PJ, Vore M. Prolactin increases hepatic Na$^+$/taurocholate co-transport activity and messenger RNA *post partum*. Biochem J. 1994;303:33–6.
36. Griffith JK, Baker ME, Rouch DA *et al*. Membrane transport proteins: implications of sequence comparisons. Curr Opin Cell Biol. 1992;4:684–95.
37. Bergwerk A, Shi X-Y, Ford AC *et al*. Immunological distribution of an organic anion transport protein (oatp) in rat liver and kidney. Hepatology. 1994;20:205A.
38. Kullak-Ublick G-A, Hagenbuch B, Stieger B, Wolkoff AW, Meier PJ. Functional characterization of the basolateral rat liver organic anion transporting polypeptide. Hepatology. 1994;20:411–16.

5
Transcellular bile acid transport

J. M. CRAWFORD

Hepatocellular processing of bile acids involves uptake from sinusoidal blood across the basolateral plasma membrane, transit through the hepatocyte, and secretion across the canalicular plasma membrane into bile. A small percentage (<5%) of secreted bile salts are newly synthesized within the hepatocyte[1]. Hepatocytes are extremely efficient in extracting bile salts from blood and secreting them into bile, accomplishing this process over a time frame of seconds to scant minutes[2]. En route, bile salts are avidly bound by cytosolic proteins such as 3α-hydroxysteroid dehydrogenase[3], and inhibition of this binding delays bile salt delivery to bile[4,5]. In this report the question of whether bile salts take any detours during their journey, into such organelles as the endoplasmic reticulum or Golgi apparatus, will be examined. Bile salts constitute two-thirds of the organic solutes in bile, and play a major role in stimulating the secretion of biliary phospholipid (primarily phosphatidylcholine) and cholesterol[1]. Moreover, biliary phosphatidylcholines appear to be derived from intracellular stores of lipid[6,7]. Thus, consideration of the intracellular processing of bile salts may also provide insights into the origins of biliary lipid.

The first glimpses of the workings of bile salts within hepatocytes came from the finding that microtubule inhibitors were capable of inhibiting bile salt secretion in intact animals or in isolated perfused liver preparations[8–10]. However, the inhibitory effects were inconstant, and difficult to interpret. An experimental model which provided consistent evidence of microtubule-dependent bile salt secretion was the depleted–reinfused rat, in which rats were subjected to overnight biliary diversion to deplete the endogenous bile salt pool, followed by reinfusion of selected bile salts at physiological rates (Fig. 1)[11]. Approximately 50% inhibition of bile salt secretion was observed when a bile salt load was imposed on the depleted liver. Increases in bile salt secretion were also inhibited about 50% when a modest bile salt load was imposed on the normal state[12]. However, the effect of microtubule inhibition on basal rates of bile salt secretion was minimal to absent. Biliary secretions of phospholipid and cholesterol were similarly inhibited[11]. More recently we have observed that the dependence on microtubule integrity of hepatic adaptation to a bile salt load increases as the hydrophobicity of the ambient bile salt pool increases[2].

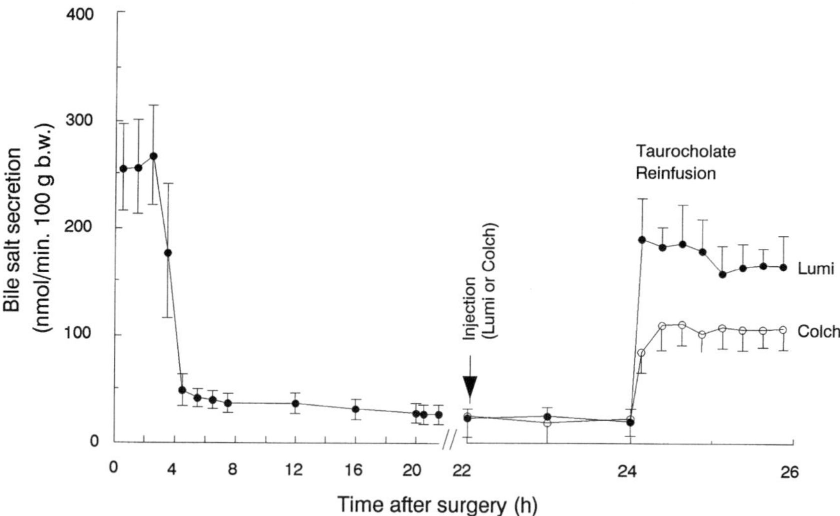

Fig. 1 Biliary secretion of bile salts following overnight biliary diversion. When intact rats fitted with intravenous and biliary catheters are subjected to overnight biliary diversion, bile salt secretion rates fall to <10% of basal values. Intravenous infusion of taurocholate (200 nmol/min per 100 g body weight) into control animals treated i.v.2 h previously (at t=22 h) with the inactive drug, lumi-colchicine (lumi, 0.12 mg/100 g), restores bile salt secretion. However, in animals pretreated with the active microtubule inhibitor, colchicine (colch), bile salt secretion is inhibited approximately 50% (Reprinted with permission from ref. 2)

Thus, microtubules are of minimal importance in maintaining bile salt secretion under steady-state conditions, but are necessary for hepatic adaptation to a bile salt load imposed on the liver. The co-dependence of phospholipid and cholesterol secretion on microtubule integrity led us initially to hypothesize that bile salts, phospholipid and possibly cholesterol moved through hepatocytes via micro-tubule-dependent vesicle trafficking[11]. While the data remain valid, key evidence will now be reviewed indicating that our initial conclusions were incorrect.

The first major observation was made by Dr Cohen and colleagues[13], who demonstrated with model membrane systems that cytosolic phosphatidylcholine-transfer protein (PC-TP) is capable of promoting the transfer of monomeric phos-phatidylcholine from the endoplasmic reticulum to the canalicular membrane. This transfer process is stimulated by physiologically relevant concentrations of bile salts, with more hydrophobic bile salts being more effective. Bile salt stimu-lation occurs as a result of bile salt interactions with the donor (endoplasmic reticulum) membrane. Realistic calculations reveal that the transfer process is capable of accounting for all biliary phosphatidylcholine secreted in bile.

A second series of important observations were made in the separate laborato-ries of Drs Apstein, Verkade and Coleman[14–18]. Bile salt-induced phospholipid secretion is absolutely dependent upon bile salt secretion as monomers into the canalicular lumen. Bile salts then appear to back-extract phospholipid from the canalicular membrane. This process is enhanced by an increased intraluminal dwell time of the bile salts[16] and by increased bile salt hydrophobicity[15]. Bile salt-induced phospholipid secretion is inhibited by the co-secretion of organic anions which bind to luminal bile salts ('uncoupling')[17–23], and by hydrophilic choleretics which sweep bile salts downstream before they can extract phospholipid[16].

Finally, kinetic studies now indicate that bile salt interactions with intracellular structures are a 'dead-end' process. In intact rats, Deroubaix and colleagues[24] have shown that radiolabelled taurocholate is rapidly secreted into bile, or partitions into a slow kinetic compartment within the liver. The partitioning increases with increasing bile salt hydrophobicity, and decreases if the more hydrophilic tauroursodeoxycholate is co-infused. This slow compartment, which represents hepatocellular organelles, does not deliver taurocholate to bile.

Drs Weinman and Maglova have conducted patch-clamping experiments with hepatocytes[25]. The rates at which fluorescent bile salts diffused into or out of a patch-clamp pipette were measured, as a function of the concentration of bile salt within the pipette. When extracellular bile salt concentration was in the low micromolar range they found that the free intracellular concentration of bile salts was submicromolar. The fluorescent bile salts were reversibly sequestered within the hepatocytes as the intracellular bile salt concentration increased, suggesting reversible interactions with intracellular structures.

Observations from a number of other laboratories have also failed to provide evidence for directed vesicular trafficking of bile salts from intracellular organelles to the canalicular pole of hepatocytes[10,26–28]. In ultrastructural studies of rapidly cryofixed hepatocytes incubated with a fluorinated bile salt analogue[29] we have found that fluorine is localized to intracellular membranes such as the endoplasmic reticulum and Golgi apparatus, but not to the lumens of these organelles or to identifiable vesicular structures. Using confocal scanning fluorescence microscopy of isolated hepatocyte couplets, the fluorescent bile salts cholyl-lysyl-fluorescein and chenodeoxycholyl-lysyl-fluorescein were found to exhibit similar rates of entry into subcellular compartments and into the bile canalicular space[30]. Inhibitors of intracellular function other than microtubule inhibitors have failed to produce inhibition of bile salt secretion in the intact liver[31].

Thus, no substantiating evidence has been obtained to indicate that intracellular membranes actually deliver bile salts to the canalicular membrane for secretion, although there is evidence for bile salt modulation of intracellular membrane function[13,32]. In fact, intracellular membrane interactions may even retard such delivery[33]. The possibility that transport systems for bile salts may be operative within intracellular compartments still remains[34–36]. Nevertheless, we must seek alternative explanations for the dependence of bile salt secretion on intracellular events.

A potential answer is forthcoming from several laboratories. Oude Elferink and colleagues have shown that the fluorescent organic anion conjugate, glutathione bimane, accumulates within intracellular vesicles when isolated hepatocytes are incubated with the non-fluorescent precursor, monochlorobimane[37]. Accumulation of fluorescence is enhanced when inhibitors of plasma membrane recycling, monensin or methylamine, are present. Hepatocytes isolated from rats which lack the appropriate multispecific organic anion transport protein do not accumulate vesicular fluorescence. Thus, it appears that canalicular membrane transport proteins are capable of recycling between the plasma membrane and interior compartments. Further evidence has been provided by Scott and Hubbard showing that canalicular membrane proteins are retrieved from the apical membrane for intracellular degradation, or are lost into bile[38]. Recent reports suggest that the delivery of bile salt transport proteins *per se* to the canalicular membrane of hepatocytes may be enhanced or diminished by the presence or absence of bile salts, respectively[39,40]. Examples of regulated plasma membrane delivery of other transport proteins have been published[41–46]. In further support of this concept are the observations that physiological modulation of bile salt flux through the liver alters the hepatic capacity for maximal canalicular bile salt secretion[47,48] and for basolateral bile salt uptake[49].

It therefore appears that an alternative explanation is possible for the experimental observations reviewed in this paper (Fig. 2). Bulk bile salt movement appears to occur via the cytosol, presumably via binding to soluble cytosolic proteins. Bile salts are then secreted as monomers into the canalicular space. Bile salts interact reversibly with intracellular membranes, where they are capable of exerting a regulatory influence, but membrane traffic *per se* does not

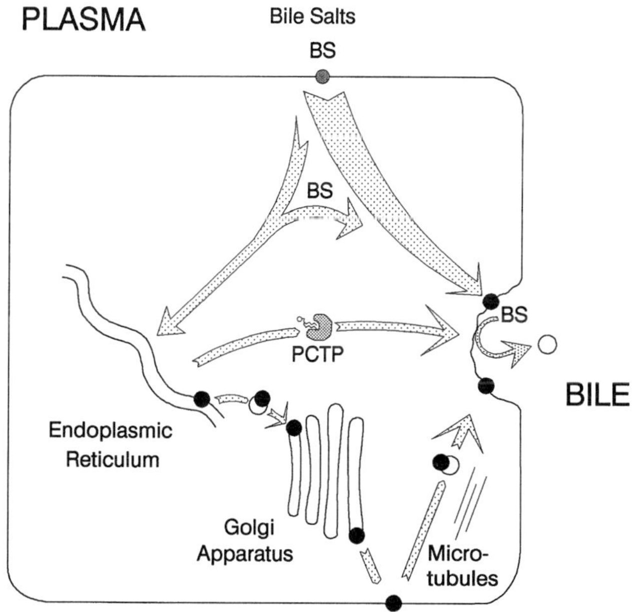

Fig. 2 Proposed intracellular transport of bile salts through hepatocytes. Bile salts are taken up across the basolateral plasma membrane from sinusoidal blood, as part of the enterohepatic circulation. The bulk of bile salts move through the cytosol to the canalicular membrane, presumably bound to soluble cytosolic proteins. Bile salts are then secreted into bile as monomers, by transport proteins located in the canalicular plasma membrane. Reversible partitioning of bile salts into intracellular compartments is thought to occur. These intracellular interactions promote the independent movement of monomeric biliary phosphatidylcholine from the endoplasmic reticulum to the canalicular membrane via phosphatidylcholite-transfer protein (PCTP), and may also promote delivery of relevant transport proteins to the canalicular membrane. Canalicular membrane proteins travel an indirect route, via the basolateral plasma membrane[50]

deliver bile salts to the canalicular membrane. Phospholipid may be delivered separately in a bile salt-stimulated fashion, via binding to phosphatidylcholine-transfer protein[13]. The hypothesis can be advanced that the relevant bile salt transport proteins are delivered to the canalicular plasma membrane in a microtubule-dependent fashion, and that delivery of these proteins is regulated by bile salt levels within hepatocytes. This hypothesis remains conjectural, but merits experimental examination in the near future.

Acknowledgements

The important contributions of the following individuals to the laboratory effort are gratefully acknowledged: Aleta R. Crawford, Deborah C. J. Strahs, Adel Z. El-Seaidy, Charles O. Mills, Victoria C. Hatch, Rebecca C. Stearns, Stephen Barnes and John J. Godleski. This work was supported by National Institutes of Health grant R01-DK39512.

References

1. Carey MC, Duane WC. Enterohepatic circulation. In: Arias IM, Boyer JL, Fausto N, Jakoby WB, Schachter D, Shafritz DA, editors. The liver: biology and pathobiology. New York: Raven Press; 1994:719–67.
2. Crawford JM, Strahs DCJ, Crawford AR, Barnes S. The role of bile salt hydrophobicity in hepatic microtubule-dependent bile salt secretion. J Lipid Res. 1994;35:1738–48.
3. Stolz A, Hammond L, Lou H, Takikawa H, Ronk M, Shively JE. cDNA cloning and expression of the human hepatic bile acid-binding protein. A member of the monomeric reductase gene family. J Biol Chem. 1993;268:10448–57.
4. Takikawa H, Stolz A, Kaplowitz N. Cyclical oxidation – reduction of the C3 position on bile acids catalyzed by rat hepatic 3α-hydroxysteroid dehydrogenase. I. Studies with the purified enzyme, isolated rat hepatocytes, and inhibition by indomethacin. J Clin Invest. 1987;80:852–60.
5. Takikawa H, Fernandez-Checa JC, Kuhlenkamp J, Stolz A, Ookhtens M, Kaplowitz N. Effect of indomethacin on the uptake, metabolism and excretion of 3-oxocholic acid: studies in isolated hepatocytes and perfused rat liver. Biochim Biophys Acta. 1991;1084:247–50.
6. Patton GM, Fasulo JM, Robins SJ. Hepatic phosphatidylcholines: evidence for synthesis in the rat by extensive reutilization of endogenous acylglycerides. J Lipid Res. 1994;35:1211–21.
7. Patton GM, Fasulo JM, Robins SJ. Origin of bile lecithins: evidence for extensive remodeling and a novel pathway of synthesis. Gastroenterology. 1993;104:A970.
8. Dubin M, Maurice M, Feldmann G, Erlinger S. Influence of colchicine and phalloidin on bile secretion and hepatic ultrastructure in the rat: possible interaction between microtubules and microfilaments. Gastroenterology. 1980;79:646–54
9. Gregory DH, Vlahcevic ZR, Prugh MF, Swell L. Mechanism of secretion of biliary lipids: role of a microtubular system in hepatocellular transport of biliary lipids in the rat. Gastroenterology. 1978;74:93–100.
10. Barnwell SG, Lowe PJ, Coleman R. The effects of colchicine on secretion into bile of bile salts, phospholipids, cholesterol and plasma membrane enzymes: bile salts are secreted unaccompanied by phospholipids and cholesterol. Biochem J. 1984;220:723–31.
11. Crawford JM, Berken CA, Gollan JL. Role of the hepatocyte microtubular system in the excretion of bile salts and biliary lipid: implications for intracellular vesicular transport. J Lipid Res. 1988;29:144–56.
12. Crawford JM, Crawford AR, Strahs DCJ. Microtubule-dependent transport of bile salts through hepatocytes: cholic vs. taurocholic acid. Hepatology. 1993;18:903–11.
13. Cohen DE, Leonard MR, Carey MC. *In vitro* evidence that phospholipid secretion into bile may be coordinated intracellularly by the combined actions of bile salts and the specific phosphatidylcholine transfer protein of liver. Biochemistry. 1994;33:9975–80.

14. Verkade JJ, Wolbers MJ, Havinga R, Uges DRA, Vonk RJ, Kuipers F. The uncoupling of biliary lipid from bile acid secretion by organic anions in the rat. Gastroenterology. 1990;99:1485–92.
15. Coleman R, Rahman K. Lipid flow in bile formation. Biochim Biophys Acta. 1992;1125:113–33.
16. Verkade HJ, Havinga R, Gerding A, Vonk RJ, Kuipers F. Mechanism of bile acid-induced biliary lipid secretion in the rat: effect of conjugated bilirubin. Am J Physiol. 1993;264:G462–9.
17. Apstein MD. Inhibition of biliary phospholipid and cholesterol secretion by bilirubin in the Sprague-Dawley and Gunn rat. Gastroenterology. 1984;87:634–8.
18. Apstein MD, Russo AR. Ampicillin inhibits biliary cholesterol secretion. Dig Dis Sci. 1985;30:253–6.
19. Monte MJ, Parslow RA, Coleman R. Inhibitory action of cyclobutyrol on the secretion of biliary cholesterol and phospholipids. Biochem J. 1990;266:165–71.
20. Bellringer ME, Steele NJ, Rahman K, Coleman R. Ampicillin inhibits the movement of biliary secretory vesicles in rat hepatocytes. Biochim Biophys Acta. 1988;941:71–5.
21. Yamashita G, Tazuma S, Horikawa K et al. Partial characterization of mechanism(s) by which sulphobromophthalein reduces biliary lipid secretion. Biochem J. 1993;291:173–7.
22. Cava F, Gonzalez J, Gonzalez-Buitrago JM, Muriel C, Jimenez R. Inhibition of biliary cholesterol and phospholipid secretion by cefmetazole. The role of vesicular transport and of canalicular events. Biochem J. 1991;275:591–5.
23. Yamashita G, Tazuma S, Kajiyama G. Effects of organic anions on biliary lipid secretion in rats. Importance of association with biliary lipid structures. Biochem J. 1992;286:193–6.
24. Deroubaix X, Coche T, Depiereux E, Feytmans E. Saturation of hepatic transport of taurocholate in rats in vivo. Am J Physiol. 1991;260:G189–96.
25. Weinman SA, Maglova LM. Free concentrations of intracellular fluorescent anions determined by cytoplasmic dialysis of isolated hepatocytes. Am J Physiol. 1994;267:G922–31.
26. Reynier MO, Hashieh IA, Crotte C, Carbuccia N, Richard B, Gerolami A. Monensin action on the Golgi complex in perfused rat liver: evidence against bile salt vesicular transport. Gastroenterology. 1992;102:2024–32.
27. Hayakawa T, Katagiri K, Hoshino M et al. Papaverine inhibits transcytotic vesicle transport and lipid excretion into bile in isolated perfused rat liver. Hepatology. 1992;16:1036–42.
28. Schubert R, Beyer K, Wolburg H, Schmidt K. Structural changes in membranes of large unilamellar vesicles after binding of sodium cholate. Biochemistry. 1986;25:5263–9.
29. Crawford JM, Barnes S, Stearns RC, Hastings CL, Godleski JJ. Ultrastructural localization of a fluorinated bile salt in hepatocytes. Lab Invest. 1994;71:42–51.
30. El-Seaidy AZ, Mills CO, Elias E, Crawford JM. Hepatocellular distribution of fluorescent bile salts: studies with confocal microscopy. Hepatology. 1993;18:136A.
31. Camogliano L, Casu A. Bile acids in bile after monensin treatment. Exp Pathol. 1989;36:37–41.
32. Crawford JM, Vinter DW, Gollan JL. Taurocholate induces pericanalicular localization of C6-NBD-ceramide in isolated hepatocyte couplets. Am J Physiol. 1991;260:G119–32.
33. LeSage GD, Schteingart CD, Hofmann AF. Effect of bile acid hydrophobicity on biliary transit time and intracellular mobility: a comparison of seven fluorescent bile acid analogues. Hepatology. 1994;20:256A.
34. Alves C, Von Dippe P, Amoui M, Levy D. Bile acid transport into hepatocyte smooth endoplasmic reticulum vesicles is mediated by microsomal epoxide hydrolase, a membrane protein exhibiting two distinct topological orientations. J Biol Chem. 1993;268:20148–55.
35. Reuben A, Allen RM. Taurocholate transport by rat liver Golgi vesicles. Gastroenterology. 1990;98:A624 (abstract).
36. Berg C, Gollan JL. Taurocholate transport by hepatocyte plasma and intracellular membranes: evaluation by 'ultra-rapid' filtration. Hepatology. 1991;14:146A.
37. Oude Elferink RPJ, Bakker CTM, Roelofsen H et al. Accumulation of organic anion in intracellular vesicles of cultured rat hepatocytes is mediated by the canalicular multispecific organic anion transporter. Hepatology. 1993;17:434–44.
38. Scott LJ, Hubbard AL. Dynamics of four rat liver plasma membrane proteins and polymeric IgA receptor. Rates of synthesis and selective loss into the bile. J Biol Chem. 1992;267:6099–106.
39. Boyer JL, McGrath JW, Ng OC. Microtubule dependent targeting of transporters to the apical membrane determines the canalicular excretion of bile acids in hepatocyte couplets. Hepatology. 1993;18:107A.
40. Crawford JM, Crawford AR. Down-regulated of hepatocyte canalicular bile salt transport by biliary diversion. Gastroenterology. 1995;108:A1053.

41. Häussinger D, Hallbrucker C, Saha N, Lang F, Gerok W. Cell volume and bile acid excretion. Biochem J. 1992;288:681–9.
42. Hallbrucker C, Lang F, Gerok W, Häussinger D. Cell swelling increases bile flow and taurocholate excretion into bile in isolated perfused rat liver. Biochem J. 1992;281:593–5.
43. Häussinger D, Saha N, Hallbrucker C, Lang F, Gerok W. Involvement of microtubules in the swelling-induced stimulation of transcellular taurocholate transport in perfused rat liver. Biochem J. 1993;291:355–60.
44. Häussinger D, Lang F, Gerok W. Regulation of cell function by the cellular hydration state. Am J Physiol Endocrinol Metab. 1994;267:E343–55.
45. Bruck R, Haddad P, Graf J, Boyer JL. Regulatory volume decrease stimulates bile flow, bile acid excretion, and exocytosis in isolated perfused rat liver. Am J Physiol. 1992;262:G806–12.
46. Bruck R, Benedetti A, Strazzabosco M, Boyer JL. Intracellular alkalinization stimulates bile flow and vesicular-mediated exocytosis in IPRL. Am J Physiol. 1993;265:G347–53.
47. Accatino L, Hono J, Koenig C, Pizarro M, Rodriguez L. Adaptive changes of hepatic bile salt transport in a model of reversible interruption of the enterohepatic circulation in the rat. J Hepatol. 1993;19:95–104.
48. Accatino L, Hono J, Maldonado M, Icarte MA, Persico R. Adaptive regulation of hepatic bile salt transport. Effect of prolonged bile salt depletion in the rat. J Hepatol. 1988;7:215–23.
49. Higgins JV, Paul JM, Dumaswala R, Heubi JE. Downregulation of taurocholate transport by ileal BBM and liver BLM in biliary-diverted rats. Am J Physiol. 1994;267:G501–7.
50. Maurice M, Schell MJ, Lardeux B, Hubbard AL. Biosynthesis and intracellular transport of a bile canalicular plasma membrane protein: studies *in vivo* and in the perfused rat liver. Hepatology. 1994;19:648–55.

6
Bile acid transport across the canalicular membrane

D. KEPPLER, R. MAYER, M. BÖHME and M. BÜCHLER

INTRODUCTION

Different proteins in the canalicular membrane of hepatocytes have been considered as transporters for bile acids and bile acid conjugates[1–9]. These include the potential-dependent transporter[1–4], the primary-active ATP-dependent transporter for bile salts such as taurocholate[5–9], and the transporter for dianionic bile salts including the glucuronic acid and sulphate conjugates of bile salts. There is accumulating evidence that the latter transporter is encoded by the multidrug resistance protein (MRP) gene[10,11]. The molecular identity of other primary-active ATP-driven export pumps in the canalicular membrane has been elucidated in part, and concerns particularly the multidrug resistance gene products[12–15]. By contrast, the molecular identity of the ATP-dependent bile salt export pump (Fig. 1) is still under investigation[16]. Strong evidence indicates that the ATP-dependent bile salt export pump, rather than potential-dependent transport, mediate the secretion of bile salts across the canalicular membrane[9,17].

RESULTS AND DISCUSSION

Decisive role of ATP-dependent canalicular bile salt secretion

The selective and potent inhibition of the canalicular ATP-dependent taurocholate export pump by cyclosporin A and its non-immuno-suppressive structural analogue PSC 833 allowed for a discrimination between potential-dependent and ATP-dependent bile salt transport[17]. The comparison of the different bile salt transport systems in hepatocyte membrane vesicles by use of the cyclosporins as tools has indicated that the ATP-dependent transporter is the only decisive one for bile salt transport across the canalicular membrane[17]. This conclusion is supported by the electrophoretic separation of the transport proteins and the demonstration that the potential-dependent transporter resides entirely in the endoplasmic reticulum[9]. Selective inhibition of ATP-dependent

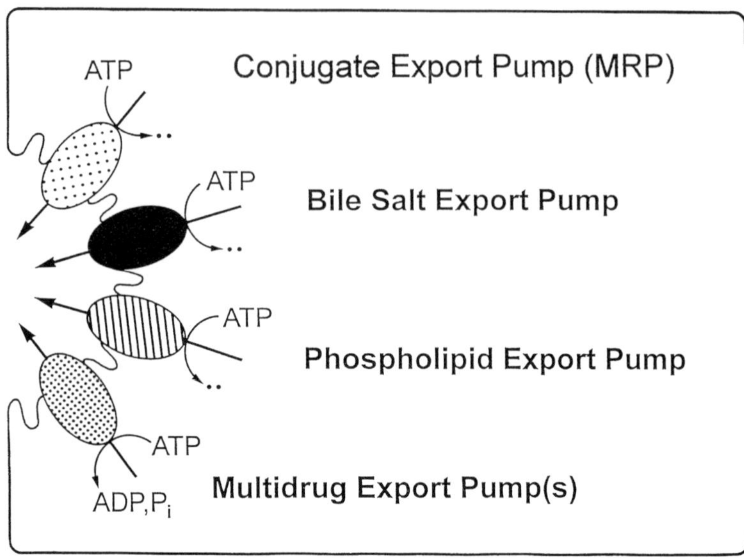

Fig. 1 ATP-dependent export pumps in the hepatocyte canalicular membrane. The multidrug resistance protein (MRP) gene-encoded conjugate export pump has recently been characterized in non-hepatic cell lines and was shown to mediate the unidirectional transport of conjugates of lipophilic compounds with anionic residues, including the glutathione *S*-conjugates leukotriene C$_4$ and *S*-(2,4-dinitrophenyl)-glutathione[10,11]. The ATP-dependent bile salt export pump has been functionally well characterized[5–8,16,17], but the corresponding gene and the molecular structure of this membrane protein are still under investigation and discussion[9,16,19–21]. The phospholipid export pump[13] which functions as a translocase[18] has been identified by disruption of the murine *mdr*2 gene[13] and further characterized by heterologous expression in yeast[18]. The multidrug export pump designates the *MDR1* gene product in humans and the *mdr1a* and *mdr1b* gene products in rodents[12]

bile salt transport by the cyclosporins strongly reduced bile flow, and this demonstrates that intrahepatic cholestasis may result from inhibition of the ATP-dependent transporter[17].

Studies on the relation of ecto-ATPase (gp 110) to the ATP-dependent bile salt export pump

ATP-dependent bile salt transport across the hepatocyte canalicular membrane has been associated with a 110 kDa glycoprotein (gp 110) which binds ATP and a photolabile bile salt derivative[5]. A similar glycoprotein was proposed as the potential-dependent bile salt transporter[3]. Sippel *et al.* have purified this 110 kDa canalicular protein, which is identical to ecto-ATPase, and demonstrated that cDNA transfection confers both bile salt efflux and ecto-ATPase activity[19–21]. Reconstitution of partially purified gp 110 into proteoliposomes resulted in an apparent ATP-dependent transport of labelled taurocholate[5]. However, the importance of a blank containing non-hydrolysable ATP analogues to replace the cosubstrate ATP was recognized only several years later[16].

More recently we studied the role of ecto-ATPase/gp 110 in ATP-dependent taurocholate transport using immunodepletion in combination with transport

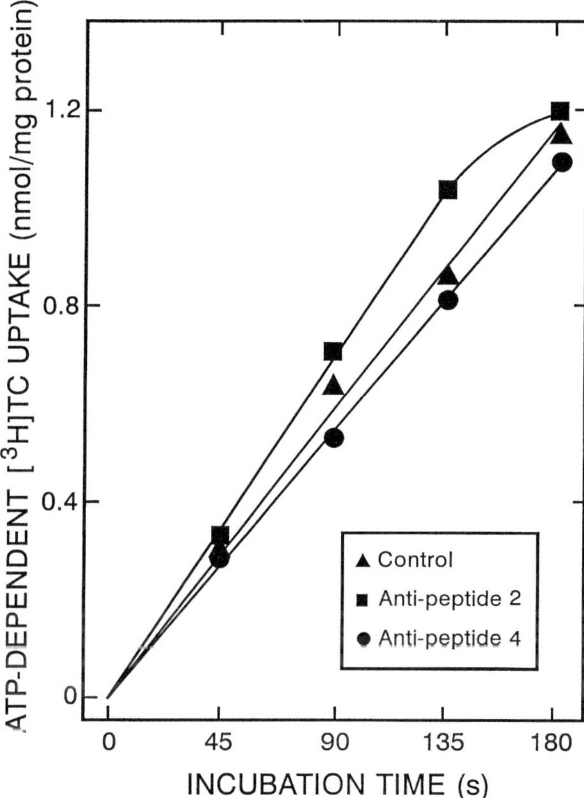

Fig. 2 ATP-dependent taurocholate (TC) transport after reconstitution of solubilized rat liver canalicular membranes into proteoliposomes with and without immunodepletion of ecto-ATPase/gp 110. Solubilization, reconstitution, and transport were performed as described recently[16]. Anti-peptide antibodies directed against the short and long isoforms of ecto-ATPase/gp 110/cell-CAM 105[22] were coupled to protein G sepharose and served to remove the major part of the solubilized ecto-ATPase/gp 110/cell-CAM 105 membrane proteins as controlled by Western blotting. The supernatants, depleted of the short isoform (anti-peptide 2) or of the long isoform (anti-peptide 4) were reconstituted into proteoliposomes. In the control, treatment was performed with protein G sepharose not coupled to antibodies. The similar transport rates indicate the lack of involvement of ecto-ATPase/gp 110/cell-CAM 105 in ATP-dependent taurocholate transport

assays in reconstituted proteoliposomes (Fig. 2). Immunoprecipitation of a major part of the solubilized ecto-ATPase did not significantly affect the rate of ATP-dependent bile salt transport by the canalicular membrane (Fig. 2). This suggests that the ATP-dependent bile salt export pump is not ecto-ATPase/gp 110. While the molecular identity of the ATP-dependent bile salt export pump remains unknown at this time, the export pump for dianionic bile salt conjugates including bile salt glucuronides has been identified as an *MRP* gene-encoded conjugate export pump[23].

Acknowledgements

This work was supported in part by the Forschungsschwerpunkt Transplantation, Heidelberg. We are grateful to Drs Werner Reutter and Oliver Baum, Berlin, for providing their peptide antisera directed against the short and long forms of gp 110/ecto-ATPase/cell-CAM 105[22].

References

1. Inoue M, Kinne R, Tran T, Arias IM. Taurocholate transport by rat liver canalicular membrane vesicles. J Clin Invest. 1984;73:659–63.
2. Meier PJ, Meier-Abt AS, Barrett C, Boyer JL. Mechanisms of taurocholate transport in canalicular and basolateral rat liver plasma membrane vesicles. J Biol Chem. 1984;259:10614–22.
3. Ruetz S, Hugentobler G, Meier PJ. Functional reconstitution of the canalicular bile salt transport system of rat liver. Proc Natl Acad Sci USA. 1988;85:6147–51.
4. Boyer JL, Graf J, Meier PJ. Hepatic transport systems regulating pH, cell volume, and the bile secretion. Annu Rev Physiol. 1992;54:415–38.
5. Müller M, Ishikawa T, Berger U et al. ATP-dependent transport of taurocholate across the hepatocyte canalicular membrane mediated by a 110-kDa glycoprotein binding ATP and bile salt. J Biol Chem. 1991;266:18920–6.
6. Adachi Y, Kobayashi H, Kurumi Y, Shouji M, Kitano M, Yamamoto T. ATP-dependent taurocholate transport by rat liver canalicular membrane vesicles. Hepatology. 1991;14:655–9.
7. Nishida T, Gatmaitan Z, Che M, Arias IM. Rat liver canalicular membrane vesicles contain an ATP-dependent bile acid transport system. Proc Natl Acad Sci USA. 1991;88:6590–4.
8. Stieger B, O'Neill B, Meier PJ. ATP-dependent bile-salt transport in canalicular rat liver plasma-membrane vesicles. Biochem J. 1992;284:67–73.
9. Kast C, Stieger B, Winterhalter KH, Meier PJ. Evidence for distinct subcellular localizations of electrogenic and ATP-dependent taurocholate transport in rat hepatocytes. J Biol Chem. 1994;269:5179–86.
10. Jedlitschky G, Leier I, Buchholz U, Center M, Keppler D. ATP-dependent transport of glutathione S-conjugates by the multidrug resistance-associated protein. Cancer Res. 1994;54:4833–6.
11. Leier I, Jedlitschky G, Buchholz U, Cole SPC, Deeley RG, Keppler D. The MRP gene encodes an ATP-dependent export pump for leukotriene C_4 and structurally related conjugates. J Biol Chem. 1994;269:27807–10.
12. Gottesman MM, Pastan I. Biochemistry of multidrug resistance mediated by the multidrug transporter. Annu Rev Biochem. 1993;62:385–427.
13. Smit JJM, Schinkel AH, Oude Elferink RPJ et al. Homozygous disruption of the murine mdr2 P-glycoprotein gene leads to complete absence of phospholipids from bile and to liver disease. Cell. 1993;75:451–62.
14. Schinkel AH, Smit JJM, Van Tellingen O et al. Disruption of the mouse mdr1a P-glycoprotein gene leads to a deficiency in the blood–brain barrier and to increased sensitivity to drugs. Cell. 1994;77:491–52.
15. Silverman JA, Raunio H, Grant TW, Thorgeirsson SS. Cloning and characterization of a member of the rat multidrug resistance (mdr) gene family. Gene. 1991;106:229–36.
16. Büchler M, Böhme M, Ortlepp H, Keppler D. Functional reconstitution of ATP-dependent transporters from the solubilized hepatocyte canalicular membrane. Eur J Biochem. 1994;224:345–52.
17. Böhme M, Müller M, Leier I, Jedlitschky G, Keppler D. Cholestasis caused by inhibition of the adenosine triphosphate-dependent bile salt transport in rat liver. Gastroenterology. 1994;107:255–65.
18. Ruetz S, Gros P. Phosphatidylcholine translocase: a physiological role for the mdr2 gene. Cell. 1994;77:1071–81.
19. Sippel CJ, Suchy FJ, Ananthanarayanan M, Perlmutter DH. The rat liver ecto-ATPase is also a canalicular bile acid transport protein. J Biol Chem. 1993;268:2083–91.
20. Sippel CJ, Fallon RJ, Perlmutter DH. Bile acid efflux mediated by the rat liver canalicular bile acid transport/ecto-ATPase protein requires serine 503 phosphorylation and is regulated by tyrosine 488 phosphorylation. J Biol Chem. 1994;269:19539–45.

21. Sippel CJ, McCollum MJ, Perlmutter DH. Bile acid transport by the rat liver canalicular bile acid transport/ecto-ATPase protein is dependent on ATP but not on its own ecto-ATPase activity. J Biol Chem. 1994;269:2800–26.
22. Baum O, Reutter W, Flanagan D *et al.* Anti-peptide antisera against cell-CAM 105 determine high molecular mass variants of the long isoform. Eur J Biochem. 1995;228:316–22.
23. Mayer R, Kartenbeck J, Büchler M, Jedlitschky G, Leier I, Keppler D. Expression of the *MRP* gene-encoded conjugate export pump in liver and its selective absence from the canalicular membrane in transport-deficient mutant hepatocytes. J Cell Biol. 1995;131:1–13.

7
The hepatic Na⁺/taurocholate cotransporter is down-regulated in experimental models of cholestasis

C. GARTUNG and J. L. BOYER

INTRODUCTION

Bile formation is an important function of the liver, which carries out various physiological processes. It includes secretion of lipophilic organic anions, such as bile acids, bilirubin, steroids and xenobiotics, and represents the only route of cholesterol excretion, either directly or by conversion of cholesterol into bile acids[1]. The flow of bile is driven by generating osmotic gradients between the portal blood, hepatocytes and bile canaliculus. Organic anions, especially bile acids and their conjugates, are the most important osmotically active solutes in bile[2]. To maintain the vectoral transport of bile acids from the portal blood to the bile canaliculus the hepatocyte is highly polarized with respect to bile acid transport systems at its basolateral (sinusoidal) and apical (canalicular) plasma membranes[3]. Functional impairment of these bile acid transporters at any level of the hepatocytes may result in cholestasis, a clinically important syndrome characterized by diminished bile flow, retention of biliary constituents in the serum, liver and others organs as well as a number of biochemical, morphological and clinical alterations associated with this syndrome[4].

HEPATIC UPTAKE OF BILE ACIDS UNDER PHYSIOLOGICAL CONDITIONS

Hepatic uptake of bile acids at the basolateral plasma membrane is the first step in hepatic bile acid transport, and is predominantly mediated by a secondary active, sodium-dependent bile acid cotransport system, which has been well characterized in various experimental systems including the isolated perfused rat liver, primary hepatocyte cell suspensions and cell cultures, and isolated basolateral liver plasma membrane preparations[5]. The basolateral Na⁺/bile acid contransporter is driven by both an inwardly directed sodium gradient, which is

maintained by the basolateral membrane ion transporter Na$^+$-K$^+$-ATPase, and the intracellular negative electrical potential, which is regulated by the outward conductance of K$^+$ via K$^+$-channels in the basolateral plasma membrane[3]. Using a functional expression cloning strategy in *Xenopus laevis* oocytes, cDNAs encoding for a sodium-dependent taurocholate cotransporting polypeptide have been cloned from rat (Ntcp) and human (NTCP) livers[6,7]. Expression of the rat Ntcp in oocytes, transiently transfected COS-7 cells or stably transfected CHO cells resulted in a strictly sodium-dependent saturable uptake of taurocholate with a similar K_m of 30–40 μmol/l, as previously determined in isolated hepatocytes and basolateral liver plasma membrane preparations[6,8,9]. Substrate specificity of Ntcp as determined in the stably transfected CHO cells included conjugated and unconjugated bile acids as well as oestrone sulphates[9]. Characterization of the native protein using antibodies raised against fusion proteins and peptides derived from the COOH-terminal part of the cloned Ntcp revealed an apparent molecular weight of 50–51 kDa, which decreased after deglycosylation of the protein to 33.5–34.5 kDa[10,11]. Deletion and site-directed mutagenesis studies showed that glycosylation of the Ntcp protein occur only at positions 5 and 11 of the potential five glycosylation sites of the polypeptide[12]. Immunofluorescent studies have confirmed the exclusive localization of Ntcp to the basolateral plasma membrane of the hepatocyte and a uniform distribution throughout the lobular gradient[10,11].

Basolateral uptake of bile acids is also mediated by a sodium-independent transport system. Recently an organic anion transporting polypeptide has been cloned from both rat (oatp) and human liver (OATP)[13,14]. In addition to a wide variety of conjugated and unconjugated bile acids the rat oatp also transports other organic anions, such as bromosulphophthalein (BSP), indocyanine and probably bilirubin[15]. Antibodies raised against a fusion protein and a peptide of oatp characterized this transporter as a glycoprotein with an apparent molecular weight of 80 kDa, which decreased to 65 kDa after deglycosylation[16]. Immunofluorescent studies showed an exclusive localization of oatp to the basolateral plasma membranes of hepatocytes[16]. Although oatp has a requirement for chloride ions when uptake of BSP is performed in the presence of albumin, the exact driving force for this transport system remains presently unknown, since uptake of BSP and bile acids can also occur at a similar maximal velocity in the absence of albumin and chloride[13].

REGULATION OF BASOLATERAL BILE ACID TRANSPORTERS

Although both the sodium-dependent and sodium-independent bile acid transport systems have been well characterized in terms of substrate specificity, driving forces and transport kinetics, little is known about their molecular regulation under physiological and pathophysiological conditions. The recent cloning of cDNAs and the development of specific antibodies, especially for Ntcp, have for the first time enabled studies to investigate the regulation of these transporters at the molecular level.

The rat liver Ntcp is only expressed in differentiated mammalian species, as it is not transcribed in mammalian hepatoma cells, dedifferentiated primary hepatocytes after 24–72 h in culture or in lower vertebrates[17,18]. Expression and activity of the Ntcp protein is also lost during hepatic regeneration following partial hepatectomy[19]. Ntcp expression and activity are developmentally regulated and appear late in gestation at day 18–21, reaching adult levels within 1–2 weeks after birth[19,20]. Prolactin increases both sodium-dependent taurocholate uptake and Ntcp mRNA in rats *post-partum*, indicating that the lactogenic hormone may be a physiological regulator of the *Ntcp* gene[21]. The differences in the degree of sodium-dependent taurocholate uptake, protein and mRNA expression of Ntcp as observed during development and in *post-partum* rats suggest that the *Ntcp* gene is regulated by both transcriptional and post-transcriptional mechanisms. Cloning of the Ntcp promotor region further indicates that bile acids might be another physiological regulator of the *Ntcp* gene[22].

EXPRESSION OF BASOLATERAL BILE ACID TRANSPORTERS DURING CHOLESTASIS

A number of preliminary reports have been published regarding the expression of the cloned Na[+]/bile acid transporter in rat models of extrahepatic and intrahepatic cholestasis[23–25]. All studies have been performed in animals, since Ntcp expression is rapidly lost in primary rat hepatocyte cultures[18] and no other suitable cell culture system has been so far established for *in-vitro* studies of Ntcp expression. In a rat model of extrahepatic cholestasis induced by bile duct ligation (CBDL), Ntcp expression was specifically down-regulated after 1 day of CBDL by 50% of sham-operated controls at the protein, mRNA and gene transcriptional levels as assessed by Western and Northern blot and a nuclear run-off assay[23]. Prolonged ligation for up to 7 days led to a virtual disappearance of the Ntcp protein, although Ntcp mRNA levels remained at 50% of controls. The disappearance of Ntcp could be confirmed by immunofluorescent microscopy, which showed no staining of either the basolateral plasma membrane or any of the intracellular compartments 7 days after CBDL. In contrast, the expression of two other integral basolateral plasma membrane proteins, the Na[+]-K[+]-ATPase and CE-9, did not decline after bile duct ligation. These results indicate that Ntcp expression is specifically down-regulated after induction of extrahepatic cholestasis, and occurs probably by both transcriptional and post-transcriptional mechanisms.

Alterations of Ntcp expression were also observed in two models of intrahepatic cholestasis[24,25]. Using endotoxin as a model of sepsis-associated cholestasis, both sodium-dependent taurocholate uptake and Ntcp mRNA declined[24]. Kinetic studies suggested that the decline in taurocholate uptake may be due to a reduction in the number of functional transporters. A similar effect on Ntcp activity could be obtained after a single injection of tumour necrosis factor alpha (TNF-α), a cytokine thought to act as the main mediator of endotoxin. In a separate study, pretreatment of rats with a monoclonal anti-TNF-α antibody prior to endotoxin injection prevented the decrease in bile flow as observed after injection of endotoxin alone[26]. Endotoxin also induces a number of other cytokines including interleukin-1 and 6 (IL-6), the latter a potent mediator of the hepatic acute-phase response after injury, but a recent study using isolated hepatocytes in culture for a maximum of 24 h showed no effect of IL-6 on Ntcp mRNA expression, although sodium-dependent taurocholate uptake was diminished by 25% in the presence of IL-6[27]. The effect of IL-6 on Na+-dependent taurocholate uptake could be explained as a secondary effect of IL-6 by inhibition of the Na+-K+-ATPase pump[27].

Oestrogen treatment of male rats is another well-characterized model of intrahepatic cholestasis, and has been used as an animal model of cholestasis in pregnancy. A number of defects have been described, including decreases in sinusoidal membrane fluidity, Na+-K+-ATPase pump activity, sodium-dependent taurocholate uptake and ATP-dependent bile acid efflux[28–30]. Studies of the time-dependent effect of ethinyl oestradiol administration in rats showed that Ntcp mRNA declined as early as 12 h after injection to 40% of controls, and remained at similar levels for up to 5 days[25]. Similar results were obtained after 5 days of oestrogen treatment, with a decline in the Ntcp mRNA by 60% and protein mass by 85% of controls[31].

In contrast to Ntcp, little is presently known about the regulation of the sodium-independent oatp under physiological or pathophysiological conditions. One preliminary study reported that the oatp mRNA expression remained unchanged in oestrogen-induced cholestasis[31].

CONCLUSIONS

The cloning of two important hepatic bile acid uptake systems enables us for the first time to examine the molecular regulation of some of the bile acid transporters, which play such an essential role in the constant formation of bile by the liver. The preliminary studies in three different models of cholestasis suggest that the basolateral sodium-dependent Ntcp seems to be maximally expressed under physiological conditions, but is rapidly down-regulated during cholestasis, irrespective of the experimental model examined. Potential regulators of the *Ntcp* gene include oestrogens, cytokines such as TNF-α, and biliary constituents such as bile acids, which are retained in the liver during cholestasis. Results of *Ntcp* gene transcriptional activity, mRNA and protein expression from these combined studies suggest that the *Ntcp* gene is both transcriptionally and post-transcriptionally regulated. Future research is needed to elucidate the exact molecular mechanisms of these regulatory processes. In addition, cloning and molecular characterization of the canalicular bile acid transporter(s), as well as understanding of the exact nature of the intracellular events of bile acid transport will be necessary to fully understand the pathophysiology of cholestasis. With a better understanding of these molecular events, more rational therapies should be able to be designed for patients with chronic cholestatic liver diseases.

References

1. Scharschmidt B. Bile formation and cholestasis. In: Zakim D, Boyer TD, editors. Hepatology: A textbook of liver disease. Philadelphia, PA: WB. Saunders; 1990:303–40.
2. Boyer JL, Graf J, Meier PJ. Hepatic transport systems regulating pH$_i$, cell volume, and bile secretion. Annu Rev Physiol. 1992;54:415–38.
3. Nathanson MH, Boyer JL. Mechanisms and regulation of bile secretion. Hepatology. 1991;14:551–66.

4. Sellinger M, Boyer JL. Physiology of bile secretion and cholestasis. In: Popper H, Schaffner F, editors. Progress in liver diseases. Philadelphia, PA: WB. Saunders; 1990:237–59.

5. Meier PJ. Transport polarity of hepatocytes. Sem Liver Dis. 1988;8:293–307.

6. Hagenbuch B, Stieger B, Foguet M, Lübbert H, Meier PJ. Functional expression cloning and characterization of the hepatocyte Na$^+$/bile acid cotransport system. Proc Natl Acad Sci USA. 1991;88:10629–33.

7. Hagenbuch B, Meier PJ. Molecular cloning, chromosomal localization, and functional characterization of a human liver Na$^+$/bile acid cotransporter. J Clin Invest. 1994;93:1326–31.

8. Boyer JL, Ng O-C, Ananthanarayanan M et al. Expression and characterization of a functional rat liver Na$^+$ bile acid cotransport system in COS-7 cells. Am J Physiol. 1994;266:G382–7.

9. Schroeder A, Hagenbuch B, Stieger B et al. The rat hepatocyte Na$^+$/taurocholate cotransporting polypeptide (Ntcp) mediates multispecific substrate transport in stably transfected chinese hamster ovary (CHO) cells. Gastroenterology. 1994;106:A979.

10. Ananthanarayanan M, Ng OC, Boyer JL, Suchy FJ. Characterization of cloned rat liver Na$^+$-bile acid cotransporter using peptide and fusion protein antibodies. Am J Physiol. 1994;267:G637–43.

11. Stieger B, Hagenbuch B, Landmann L, Höchli M, Schroeder A, Meier PJ. In-situ localization of the hepatocytic Na$^+$/taurocholate cotransporting polypeptide in rat liver. Gastroenterology. 1994;107:1781–7.

12. Stieger B, Hagenbuch B, Cornacchia L, Schroeder A, Landmann L, Meier PJ. Molecular properties of the Na$^+$-dependent taurocholate cotransporter polypeptide (Ntcp) of rat liver. Hepatology. 1993;18:143A.

13. Jacquemin E, Hagenbuch B, Stieger B, Wolkoff AW, Meier PJ. Expression cloning of a rat liver Na$^+$-independent organic anion transporter. Proc Natl Acad Sci USA. 1994;91:133–7.

14. Kullak-Ublick G-A, Hagenbuch B, Stieger B, Schteingart CD, Hofmann AF, Meier PJ. Cloning and functional characterization of a human liver basolateral organic anion transporting polypeptide (OATP). Hepatology. 1994;19:871.

15. Kullak-Ublick G-A, Hagenbuch B, Stieger B, Wolkoff AW, Meier PJ. Functional characterization of the basolateral rat liver organic anion transporting polypeptide. Hepatology. 1994;20:411–16.

16. Bergwerk A, Shi X-Y, Ford AC et al. Immunologic distribution of an organic anion transport protein (oatp) in rat liver and kidney. Hepatology. 1994;20:205A.

17. Boyer JL, Hagenbuch B, Ananthanarayanan M, Suchy FJ, Stieger B, Meier PJ. Phylogenic and ontogenic expression of hepatocellular bile acid transport. Proc Natl Acad Sci USA. 1993;90:435–8.

18. Liang D, Hagenbuch B, Stieger B, Meier PJ. Parallel decrease of Na$^+$-taurocholate cotransport and its encoding mRNA in primary cultures of rat hepatocytes. Hepatology. 1993;18:1162–6.

19. Green RM, Lipin AI, Pelletier EM et al. Hepatic regeneration is associated with a marked reduction in mRNA expression of the basolateral Na$^+$-taurocholate transporter. Gastroenterology. 1994;106:A901.

20. Hardikar W, Ananthanarayanan M, Sippel CJ, Suchy FJ. Developmental regulation of hepatic bile acid transport systems. Hepatology. 1993;18:143A.

21. Ganguly TC, Liu Y, Hyde JF, Hagenbuch B, Meier PJ, Vore M. Prolactin increases hepatic Na$^+$/taurocholate co-transport activity and messenger RNA post partum. Biochem J. 1994;303:33–6.

22. Karpen S, Ananthanarayanan M, Hagenbuch B, Meier PJ, Suchy FJ. Functional analysis of the rat liver sinusoidal Na$^+$-dependent bile acid transporter gene promotor. Gastroenterology. 1993;104:A925.

23. Gartung C, Ananthanarayanan M, Rahman MA, Stolz A, Suchy FJ, Boyer JL. Cholestasis induces down-regulation of the sodium-dependent bile acid cotransporter and cytosolic binding proteins following bile duct ligation in the rat. Hepatology. 1993;18:139A.

24. Mosley RH, Wang W, Takeda H, Bully T, Shick L, Kacholiya S. Endotoxin and tumor necrosis factor α inhibition of sinusoidal and canalicular bile acid transport – functional and molecular studies. Hepatology. 1993;18:136A.

25. Simon FR, Fortune J, Iwahashi M, Sutherland E. Dual mechanisms involved in early pathogenesis of ethinyl estradiol cholestasis. Hepatology. 1994;19:124I.

26. Whiting JF, Rosenbluth AB, Narciso JP, Gollan JL. Tumor necrosis factor-α inhibits taurocholate uptake by hepatocytes: implications for the pathogenesis of endotoxin-induced cholestasis. Gastroenterology. 1991;100:A811.

27. Green RM, Whiting JF, Rosenbluth AB, Beier D, Gollan JL. Interleukin-6 inhibits hepatocyte taurocholate uptake and sodium–potassium–adenosinetriphosphate activity. Am J Physiol. 1994;267:G1094–1100.

28. Reyes H, Simon FR. Intrahepatic cholestasis of pregnancy: an estrogen-related disease. Sem Liver Dis. 1993;13:289–301.

29. Berr F, Simon FR, Reichen J. Ethynylestradiol impairs bile salt uptake and Na-K pump function of rat hepatocytes. Am J Physiol. 1984;247:G437–43.

30. Bossard R, Stieger B, O'Neill B, Fricker G, Meier PJ. Ethinylestradiol treatment induces multiple canalicular membrane transport alterations in rat liver. J Clin Invest. 1993;91:2714–20.

31. Kupferschmidt H, Hagenbuch B, Stieger B, Kraehenbühl St, Meier PJ. Ethinylestradiol induces differential effects on various transporter mRNA and protein levels in rat liver. Hepatology. 1994;20:175A.

Section III
New concepts of bile acid-induced hepatotoxicity and bile secretion

8
Effect of bile salts on biomembranes

S. GÜLDÜTUNA, G. ZIMMER and U. LEUSCHNER

Bile salts are amphoteric molecules with detergent properties. It has been suggested that toxic bile salts may play a pathogenic role in liver diseases[1–4]. The apolar α-dihydroxy-bile salts are cytotoxic and induce cholestasis and necrosis of the liver[5–8].

In liver perfusion studies with chenodeoxycholate (CDC), an α-dihydroxy-bile salt, progressive damage to the liver was observed. Following perfusion with 0.01 mmol/l CDC liver plasma membranes were isolated and an inhibition of the Na-K-ATPase was detected (Fig. 1). Na-K-ATPase is localized in the basolateral domain of the plasma membrane. Alterations in the lipid membrane structure could induce an inhibition of this enzyme accompanied by cholestasis[9]. At concentrations of 0.3 mmol/l CDC induced morphological alterations of the plasma membranes (Fig. 2). Electron microscopy revealed bleb formation at the basolateral membrane and destruction of the canalicular domain. Increasing the CDC concentrations of 0.5 mmol/l led to damage of cell organelles, e.g. swelling of mitochondria (Fig. 3). Ursodeoxycholate (UDC), a more polar bile salt, had no toxic effects on the liver.

Since the initial effects of bile salt toxicity were observed on hepatocyte plasma membranes we focused our investigations on alterations in the plasma membrane. Alterations in the molecular structure of membranes can be detected using sensitive methods such as electron paramagnetic resonance spectroscopy (EPR). We therefore investigated alterations in the lipid structure of the membrane with this technique. Specimens were labelled with a nitroxide stable radical, attached to a stearic acid molecule. The spin labels 16-DSA and 5-DSA provide information on the polarity (a_N) and molecular motion (Fig. 4) in their environments[10,11]. 16-DSA reports on the apolar domain and 5-DSA on the interphase (Fig. 5) of the membrane[12].

Apolar bile salts increased the polarity of the membrane[13,14]. Figure 6 shows three different plasma membranes: erythrocyte, canalicular and basolateral liver plasma membranes. Addition of CDC induced an increase in the polarity of the membrane lipid domain. The extent of the change in the polarity depends on the cholesterol concentration of the membrane. In membranes low in cholesterol the polarity increased, whereas membranes with higher cholesterol content were

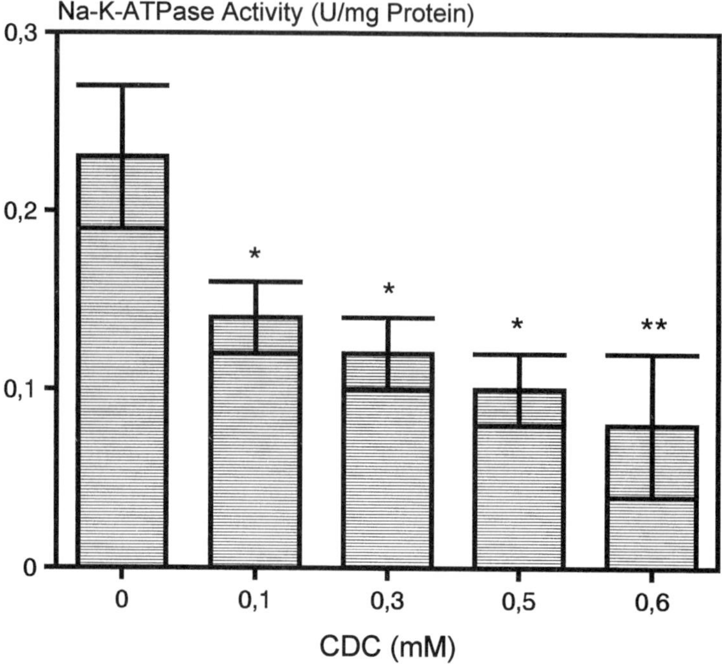

Fig. 1 Activity of the Na-K-ATPase in isolated liver plasma membranes after perfusion of the liver with different concentrations of CDC for 90 min. *$p < 0.05$, **$p < 0.01$ versus control

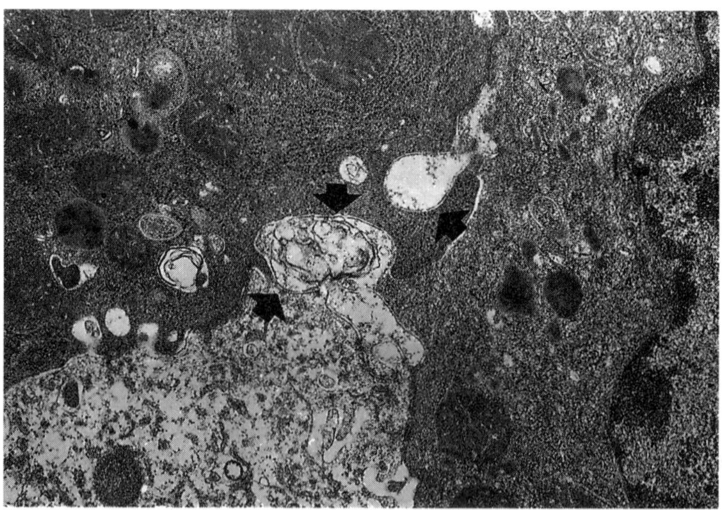

Fig. 2 Morphological alterations of the liver plasma membranes detected by electron microscopy after perfusion with 0.3 mmol/l CDC for 90 min. Notice the destruction at the canalicular domain (marked with an arrow)

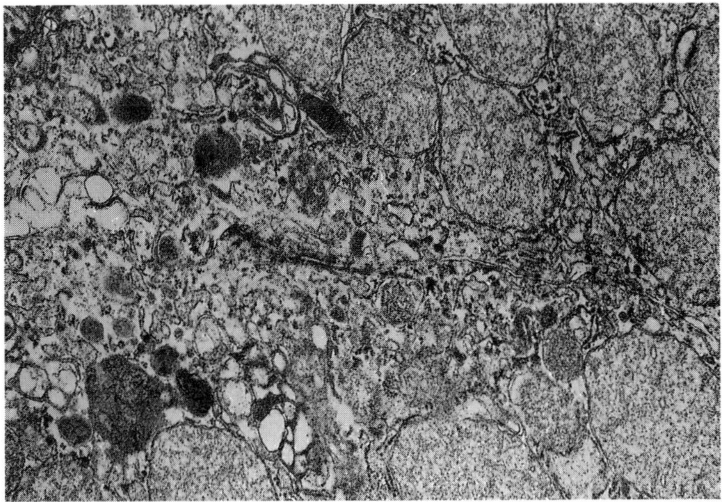

Fig. 3 Morphological alterations of the liver detected by electron microscopy after perfusion with 0.5 mmol/l CDC for 90 min. Notice the swelling of the mitochondria

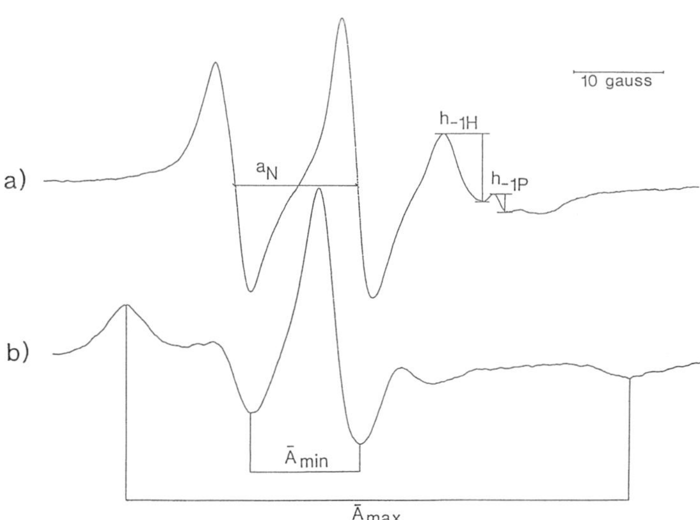

Fig. 4 EPR spectra of (**a**) 16-DSA and (**b**) 5-DSA incorporated into erythrocyte membranes. Polarity estimations: a_N assesses the water penetration into biological membranes. h_{-1P}/h_{-1H} is a parameter for measuring the amounts of spin label molecules in polar and apolar environments. Order parameters: $\bar{A}_{min}$ and $\bar{A}_{max}$ indicate the deviance of the axis of rapid rotation of spin label from the bilayer perpendicular

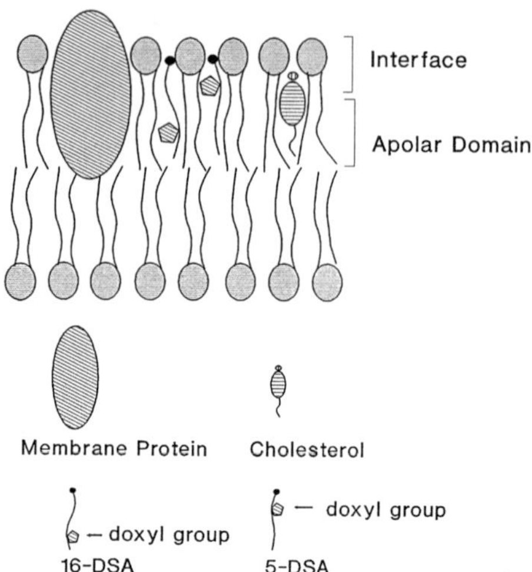

Fig. 5 Localization of 5-DSA and 16-DSA in the lipid bilayer

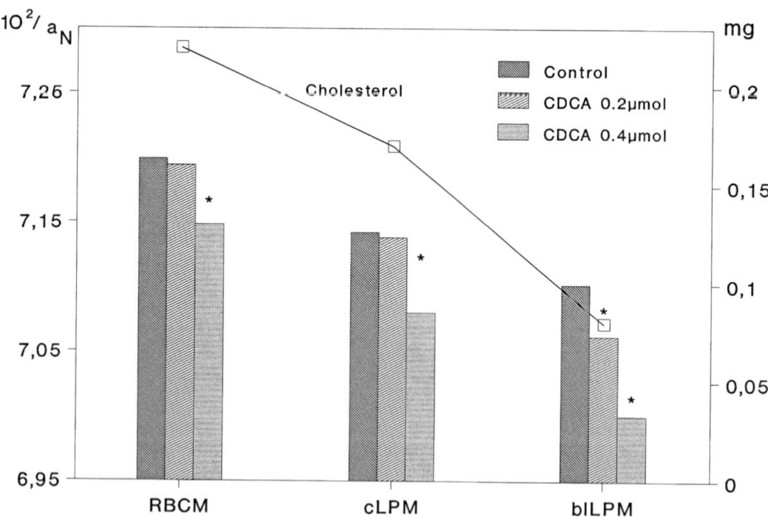

Fig. 6 Correlation of cholesterol concentration (mg/mg membrane protein) in different membrane fractions and sensitivity to CDC damage, shown by changes in membrane polarity (a_N). Membranes were labelled with 16-DSA. *$p < 0.001$ versus control

not affected. However, higher concentrations of CDC also induced an increase in the polarity of erythrocyte (ERM) and canalicular liver plasma membranes (cLPM), which have a higher cholesterol content than basolateral liver plasma membranes. Thus, membranes with low cholesterol concentration are more sensitive to apolar bile salts.

The increase in membrane permeability and polarity depends on the hydrophobicity of the bile salt molecule. The greatest increase in membrane polarity is induced by deoxycholate (DC), followed by CDC. The conjugates had a milder effect on membrane polarity. UDC decreased the polarity in the hydrophobic region of the membrane, whereas its conjugates did not affect this apolar domain (Fig. 7). An increase in membrane polarity is due to a perturbation in membrane structure, which permits water to permeate deeper into the membrane interior[11,12,14].

The increase in membrane polarity caused by toxic bile salts is accompanied by an increase in membrane permeability. Efflux of carboxyfluorescein (CF) or inulin from vesicles made out of model membranes are standard methods to investigate membrane permeability[15–17]. CF efflux was induced even by concentration of 0.05 mmol/l CDC[15], and similar results were obtained for inulin release[17]. The CF efflux depends on the cholesterol content of the membrane. In order to induce the same CF efflux in membranes with increased cholesterol content the CDC concentration has to be increased (Fig. 8). However, cholesterol contents (Fig. 8) > 30% have no additional stabilizing effect against CDC-induced permeability changes. Concentrations of 50% cholesterol destabilized the membranes and the permeability is increased compared to LUV (large unilamellar vesicles) without cholesterol (LUV with 100% egg yolk lecithin (EYL)). Thus the stabilizing effect of cholesterol is limited and more than 40% destabilizes the membranes. Alterations in membrane polarity and fluidity could also alter membrane function like the inhibition of membrane-bound enzymes[9,18], or damage the whole cell[19–21].

The influence of bile salts on membrane lipid structure is due to their binding to the membrane, and depends on the hydrophobicity of the bile salts[22]. The greater the hydrophobicity, the stronger the binding to the membrane. Schubert et al.[16,17] investigated the binding equilibria of bile salts to model membranes (LUV) by means of Scatchard plots. The highest association constant (K_a) is

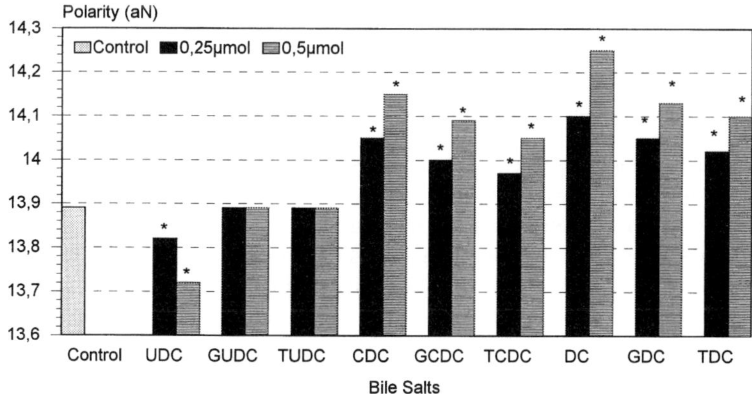

Fig. 7 Effect of different bile salts (μmol/mg membrane protein) on the polarity of erythrocyte membranes. The polarity (a_N) of the apolar domain of the membranes was detected with 16-DSA. *$p < 0.01$ versus control

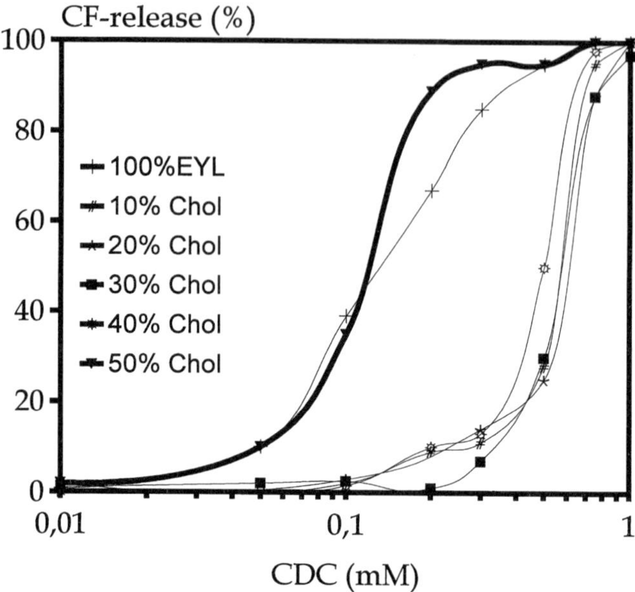

Fig. 8 Carboxyfluorecein efflux of large unilamellar vesicles with different cholesterol concentrations induced by CDC; incubation time 60 s

found with CDC, followed by UDC and cholate (C). The association constant depends on the lipid composition of the membrane. Increasing the membrane cholesterol content decreases the association constant. Thus cholesterol hampered the binding of bile salts to phospholipid membranes. The number of lipid molecules which are associated with one bile salt molecule at low bile salt concentrations could also be calculated by means of Scatchard plots. Cholate is associated with six lipid molecules, CDC with three UDC with 16. The number of lipid molecules per bile acid molecule increases with increasing cholesterol content of the membrane.

After binding to membranes, bile salts pass through the membrane. The trans-bilayer movement of bile salts has been measured with pyranin, a pH-sensitive fluorescent molecule[23]. Passing the membrane bile salts drop the pH, e.g. DC induces a pH decrease from 7.4 to 6.9. Thus the pK of the bile salts is different in the outer and inner leaflet of the membrane. The diffusion time of CDC and DC is very short; $t_{\frac{1}{2}}$ is less than 1 s, whereas that of cholate (C), a more polar bile salt, is 10–15 times longer. NMR studies have shown that the diffusion time of C is more than 50 times longer than that of α-dihydroxy-bile salts; conjugated bile salts do not pass through the membrane[24].

The diffusion potential of bile salts depends on their hydrophobicity. Upon entering the outer leaflet of the membrane, bile salts increase the polarity[14], and decrease the order by forming polar compartments in the outer leaflet. The increase in the energetic potential (ΔG) between the outer and inner leaflet of the membrane, increases the diffusion potential. This could induce a redistribution of bile salt molecules, leading to a transient pore formation in the membrane (Fig. 9), which increases permeability of the membrane[16,17].

Increasing the bile salt concentration of α-dihydroxy-bile salts to the critical micellar concentration (CMC), induced solubilization of model membranes into bile salt/lipid mixed disc micelles[25, 26]. Prior to onset of membrane solubilization vesicle size increased, indicating that the bile salt/lipid ratio increased. The membrane solubilization induced by CDC occurs at concentrations of 1.25 mmol/l in 100% EYL vesicles. With increased membrane cholesterol content the CDC concentration has to be increased (Fig. 9). UDC, a hydrophilic

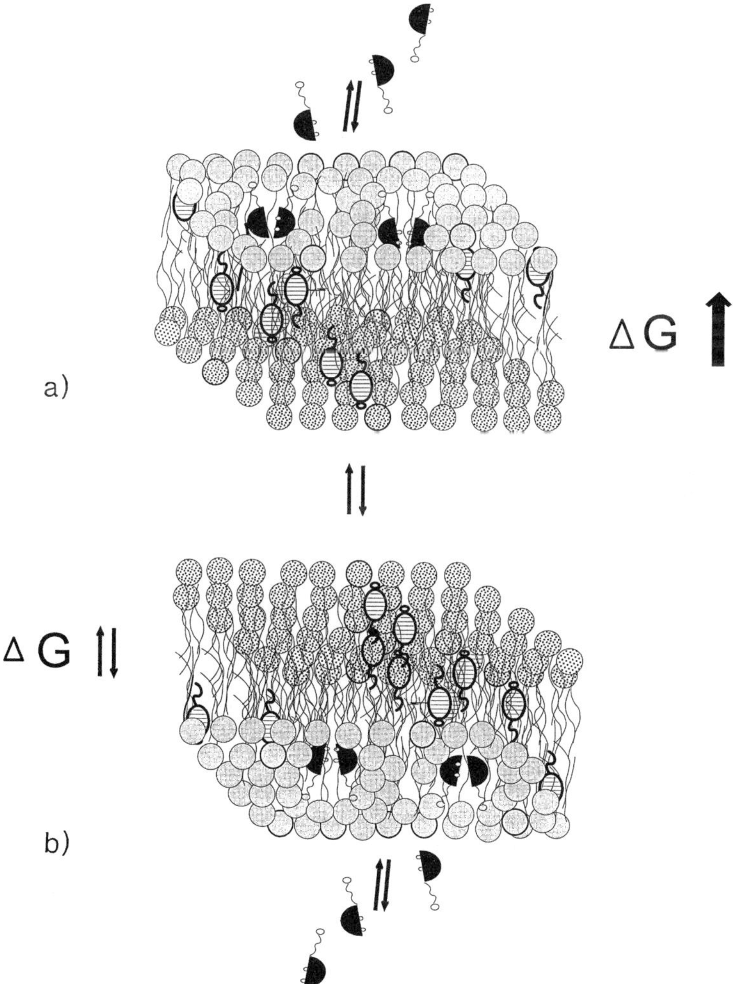

Fig. 9 Membrane diffusion of bile salts showing the induction of pore formation in the membrane. (**a**) Insertion of CDC into the outer leaflet of a model membrane, increasing the polarity and decreasing the order of membrane lipids. (**b**) Diffusion of CDC to the inner leaflet of a model membrane

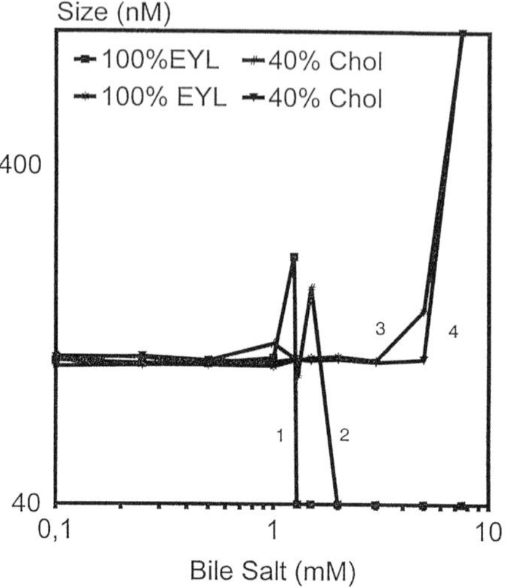

Fig. 10 Effect of CDC (1,2) and UDC (3,4) on the size (measured by laser light scattering) of large unilamellar vesicles with different cholesterol contents

3α-7β-dihydroxy-bile salt, induced vesicle fusion above the CMC to multi-lamellar aggregates larger than 1 μm (Fig. 10), probably by forming apolar clusters of UDC on the surface of the vesicles similar to cholesterol[27].

In *in-vitro* and *in-vivo* experiments polar bile salts prevented the damage induced by apolar bile salts[28–33]. The increase in membrane permeability induced by CDC was reduced by simultaneous incubation with UDC[33]. In EPR experiments UDC prevented the increase in membrane polarity caused by apolar bile salts[14]. Since this protective effect could be observed in both erythrocyte and basolateral liver plasma membranes, this phenomenon is not specific for hepatocyte membranes. The mechanism of membrane protection by UDC could be induced by molecular interaction of the bile salt molecules in the buffer or by direct membrane protection. In preincubation experiments non-membrane-bound UDC was removed and membranes were then post-incubated with CDC, but UDC still prevented the increase in membrane polarity. Thus the membrane stabilization of UDC could be a direct effect on the membrane.

The possible arrangements of bile salt molecules in the membrane bilayers are shown in Fig. 11. NMR experiments have shown that α-dihydroxyl-bile salts are inserted as dimers into the membrane[34], whereas cholate molecules lie flat on the membrane surface[35]. In our EPR experiments with different lipid labels we found that UDC induced a decrease of polarity in the apolar part of the membrane, and the conjugates induced a decrease of polarity in the membrane interphase[14]. We concluded from these results that the steroid nucleus of UDC is located in the apolar domain and that of the conjugates in the interphase (Fig. 12).

The binding site of UDC is similar to that of cholesterol[36]. In some ways UDC mimics the effects of cholesterol on phospholipid membranes[27], e.g. UDC

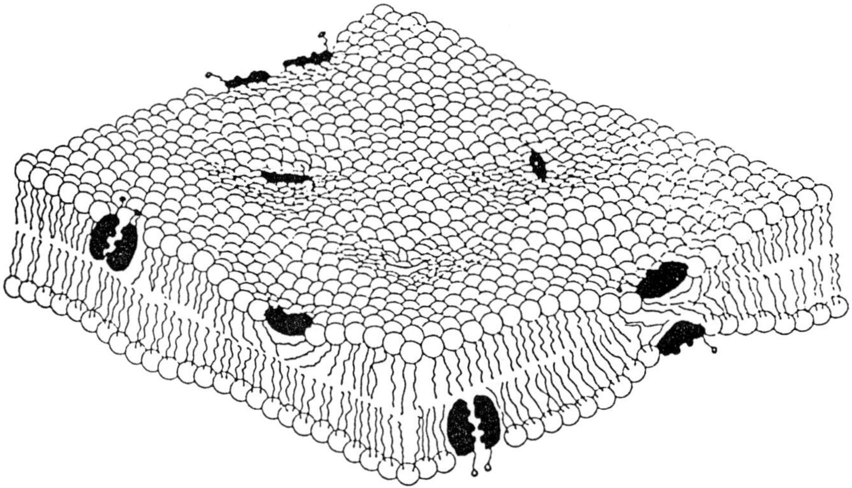

Fig. 11 Scheme indicating the different possible localizations of bile salt molecules in the lipid bilayer (A. F. Hofmann, *The Liver*, Raven Press, 1994)

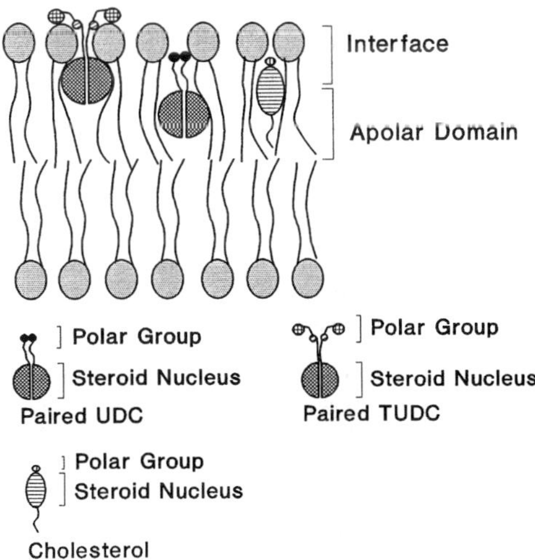

Fig. 12 Localization of UDC and TUDC in the plasma membrane as detected by EPR technique

decreases the polarity of the membranes as does cholesterol[14,37]. The enthalpy of the phase transition of phospholipid membranes is also reduced by UDC[38] in a fashion similar to cholesterol[36,37]. The similarities between UDC and cholesterol concerning their interaction with phospholipid membranes may be of relevance of the therapeutic effect of UDC.

References

1. Attili AF, Angelico M, Cantafora A, Alvaro D, Capocaccia L. Bile acid induced liver toxicity: relation to the hydrophobic balance of bile acids. Med Hypoth. 1986;19:57–69.
2. Carey JB. Bile salts and hepatobiliary diseases. In: Schiff L, editor. Diseases of the liver Philadelphia, PA: Lippincott; 1960:103–27.
3. Greim H, Trülzsch D, Czygan P *et al.* Mechanism of cholestasis. 6. Bile acids in human livers with or without biliary obstruction. Gastroenterology. 1972;63:846–50.
4. Güldütuna S, Leuschner M, Wunderlich N *et al.* Cholic acid and ursodeoxycholic acid therapy in primary biliary cirrhosis. Changes in bile acid pattern and their correlation with liver function. Eur J Clin Pharmacol. 1993;45:221–5.
5. Drew R, Priestly BG. Choloretic and cholestatic effects of infused bile salts in the rat. Experientia. 1978;35:809.
6. Dryska H, Chen T, Salen G, Mosbach EH. Toxicity of chenodeoxycholic acid in the rhesus monkey. Gastroenterology. 1975;69:333–7.
7. Miyai K, Price VM, Fisher MM. Bile acid metabolism in mammals. Ultrastructural studies on intrahepatic cholestasis induced by lithocholic and chenodeoxycholic acids in the rat. Lab Invest. 1971;24:292–302.
8. Miyazaki K, Nakayama F, Koga A. Effect of chenodeoxycholic and ursodeoxycholic acid on isolated adult human hepatocytes. Dig Dis Sci 1984;29:1123–30.
9. Keeffe EB, Scharschmidt BF, Blankenship NB, Ockner RK. Studies on relationship among bile flow, liver plasma membrane NaK-ATPase and membrane viscosity in the rat. J Clin Invest. 1979;64:1590–8.
10. Griffith OH, Jost PC. Lipid spin labels in biological membranes. In: Berliner LJ, editor. Spin labeling, theory and applications. New York: Academic Press; 1976;453–523.
11. Keith AD, Sharnoff M, Cohn GE. A summary and evaluation of spin labeling used as probes for biological membrane structure. Biochim Biophys Acta. 1973;300:379–419.
12. Marsh D. Electron spin resonance: spin labels. In: Grell E, editor. Membrane spectroscopy. Molecular biology, biochemistry and biophysics, 31. Berlin-New York: Springer; 1981:51–142.
13. Güldütuna S, Kurtz W, Pelekanos C, Zimmer G, Leuschner U. Rank of toxicity for different bile salts measured with electron spin resonance (ESR). Gastroenterology. 1989;96:A604 (abstract).
14. Güldütuna S, Zimmer G, Imhof M, Bhatti S, You T, Leuschner U. Molecular aspects of membrane stabilization by ursodeoxycholate. Gastroenterology. 1993;104:1736–44.
15. Gülütuna S, Weiß A, Deisinger B *et al.* The effect of chenodeoxycholate (CDC) on large unilamellar vesicles (LUV) with variable cholesterol concentration. Gastroenterology. 1994;106:A902.
16. Schubert R, Beyer K, Wolburg H, Schmidt KH. Structural changes in membranes of large unilamellar vesicles after binding of sodium cholate. Biochemistry. 1986,25:5263–9.
17. Schubert R, Schmidt KH. Structural changes in vesicle membranes and mixed micelles of various lipid compositions after binding of different bile salts. Biochemistry. 1988;27:8787–94.
18. Rosario J, Sutherland E, Zaccaro L, Simon FR. Ethinylestradiol administration selectively alters liver sinusoidal membrane lipid fluidity and protein composition. Biochemistry. 1988;27:3339–46.
19. Owen JS. Extrahepatic cell membrane lipid abnormalities and cellular dysfunction in liver diseases. Drugs 1990;40 (Suppl):73–83.
20. Schachter D. Fluidity and function of hepatocyte plasma membranes. Hepatology. 1984;4:140–51.
21. Smith DJ, Gordon ER. Membrane fluidity and cholestasis. J Hepatol. 1987;5:362–5.
22. Armstrong MJ, Carey MC. The hydrophobic–hydrophilic balance of bile salts. Inverse correlation between reverse high performance liquid chromatographic mobilities and micellar cholesterol-solubilizing capacities. J Lipid Res. 1982;23:70–80.
23. Kamp F, Hamilton JA. Movement of fatty acid analogues and bile acids across phospholipid bilayers. Biochemistry. 1993;32:11074–86.
24. Cabral DJ, Small DM, Lilly HS, Hamilton JA. Transbilayer movement of bile acids in model membranes. Biochemistry. 1987,26:1801–4.
25. Mazer NA, Kwasnik RF, Carey MC, Benedek GB. Quasielastic light spectroscopic studies of aqueous bile salt–lecithin and bile salt–lecithin–cholesterol solutions. Micell, Solubil, Microencaps. 1976;1:382–402.

26. Small DM. The physical chemistry of cholanic acids in the bile acids. In: Nair PP, Kritchevsky D, editors. Chemistry, Physiology and metabolism. Vol. 1, Chemistry. New York: Plenum Press; 1971:249.

27. Güldütuna S, Weiß A, Deisinger B, *et al.* Ursodeoxycholate (UDC) mimics the membrane stabilizing effect of cholesterol on large unilamellar vesicles (LUV). Gastroenterology. 1994;106:A902.

28. Heuman DM, Pandak WM, Hylemon PB, Vlahcevic ZR. Conjugates of ursodeoxycholate protect against cytotoxicity of more hydrophobic bile salts: *in vitro* studies in rat hepatocytes and human erythrocytes. Hepatology. 1991;14:920–6.

29. Kanai S, Kitani K. Glycoursodeoxycholate (GU) is as effective as tauroursodeoxycholate (TU) in preventing the taurocholate induced cholestasis in the rat. Hepatology. 1983;3:810 (abstract).

30. Kitani K, Ohta M, Kanai S. Tauroursodeoxycholate prevents biliary protein excretion induced by other bile salts in the rat. Am J Physiol. 1985;248:G407–17.

31. Kitani K, Kanai S. Effect of ursodeoxycholate on the bile flow in the rat. Life Sci. 1982;31:1973–85.

32. Kitani K, Kanai S. Tauroursodeoxycholate prevents taurocholate induced cholestasis in the rat. Life Sci. 1982;30:515–23.

33. Güldütuna S, Deisinger B, Weiß A, Sippos P, Freisleben HJ, Leuschner U. Cholesterol-like effects of ursodeoxycholate (UDC) on large unilamellar vesicles (LUV). Hepatology. 1994;20,A262.

34. Saito H, Sugimoto Y, Tabeta R *et al.* Incorporation of bile acids of low concentration into model and biological membranes studied by ^{2}H and ^{31}P NMR. J Biochem (Tokyo). 1983;94:1877–87.

35. Ulmius J, Lindblom G, Wennerström H *et al.* Molecular organization in the liquid-crystalline phases of lecithin–sodium cholate–water systems studied by nuclear magnetic resonance. Biochemistry. 1982;21:1553–60.

36. Yeagle PL. Cholesterol and the cell membrane. Biochim Biophys Acta. 1985;822:267–87.

37. El-Sayed MY, Guion TA, Fayer MD. Effect of cholesterol on visoelastic properties of dipalmitoylphosphatidylcholine multibilayers as measured by laser-induced ultrasonic probe. Biochemistry. 1986;25:4825–30.

38. Güldütuna S, Deisinger B, Weiß A, Sippos P, Freisleben HJ, Leuschner U. Ursodeoxycholate (UDC) mimics the effect of cholesterol on the phase transition of egg yolk lecithin (EYL). Hepatology. 1994;20:A1029.

9
Apoptosis – an alternative mechanism of bile salt hepatotoxicity

T. PATEL, J. SPIVEY, J. VADAKEKALAM and G. J. GORES

INTRODUCTION

The accumulation of toxic bile salts within hepatocytes has been postulated as a mechanism of hepatotoxicity during chronic cholestasis[1,2]. Indeed, many hydrophobic bile salts are directly toxic to hepatocytes. In addition recent data indicate that the bile salt ursodeoxycholate may ameliorate human cholestatic liver disease by displacing toxic bile salts from the human bile salt pool[3]. The study of the cellular mechanisms of lethal bile salt injury is therefore highly pertinent and relevant to understanding the pathogenesis of human cholestatic liver disease.

Lethal cellular injury can arise by one or two general mechanisms: apoptosis or necrosis[4]. Cell necrosis is injury that occurs due to a toxic or environmental insult, and is characterized by loss of plasma membrane integrity[5]. In contrast, apoptosis is morphologically defined cell death and is characterized by nuclear and cellular fragmentation with subsequent break-up of the cell into membrane-bound fragments containing structurally intact organelles referred to as apoptotic bodies[6]. The plasma membrane remains intact during apoptosis, thereby preventing the release of intracellular constituents. During apoptosis, cleavage of DNA at internucleosomal regions into multiples of 180–200 base pairs generates a ladder-like pattern on agarose gel electrophoresis[7]. Although originally recognized as a form of physiological cell death, it is now recognized that apoptotic cell death can also result from a toxic, environmental insult[4,8].

Previous studies on the mechanism of bile-salt-induced injury have focused on cell injury by necrosis. Bile-salt-induced lethal hepatocellular injury has been attributed to direct membrane damage due to the detergent-like properties of hydrophobic bile salts, as well as resulting from alterations in cytosolic free Ca^{2+} or cellular ATP[9–13]. These forms of injury culminate in the loss of plasma membrane integrity and cell necrosis. It has recently been appreciated that identical toxins can cause cell injury by both necrosis and apoptosis, with low concentrations of the toxin causing apoptosis and high concentrations resulting in necrosis. These observations suggest that, since high concentrations of bile salts cause necrosis, lower concentrations may induce apoptosis. Indeed, the typical sequelae of apoptotic cell death, such as cell drop-out and acidophilic (apoptotic) bodies, are commonly observed histopathological features of cholestatic liver disease, whereas widespread cell necrosis is not[14]. These observations led us to investigate whether cell death by apoptosis was a mechanism of bile-salt-induced hepatocellular injury. Our studies are summarized in this chapter. First we established that toxic bile salts induce apoptosis in hepatocytes by a mechanism involving endonuclease activity. Next we evaluated the *in-vitro* cation dependence of hepatocyte nuclear endonuclease activity and the effects of bile salts on cellular divalent cation concentrations. We then studied the relationship between bile salt hydrophobicity and injury by both apoptosis and necrosis. Finally we determined the effect of ursodeoxycholate and its conjugates on cytoprotection from apoptosis.

METHODS AND MATERIALS

Hepatocyte isolation and culture

Hepatocytes were isolated from adult male Sprague-Dawley rats (250–350 g) and cultured on glass coverslips as previously described in detail[15].

Assessment of apoptosis

Apoptosis was quantitated by identifying nuclear changes indicative of apoptosis using the DNA binding dye acridine orange and fluorescence microscopy as previously described[15]. Cultured hepatocytes were stained with 5 μmol/l acridine orange. The coverslips were transferred to a glass slide and viewed under a fluorescence microscope at a magnification of 250 (Carl Zeiss Inc., Thornwood, NY). Acridine orange fluorescence was visualized using 450–490 nm excitation filters and 515–565 nm emission filters, respectively. At least 300 cells were counted. Fluorescent-stained nuclei were considered to be fragmented if at least three separate fragments of condensed chromatin were identified in a cell.

Assessment of cell necrosis

Necrosis was determined in cell suspensions from the total fluorescence of propidium iodide as previously described[16].

Bile salt uptake

Bile salt uptake was determined by incubating hepatocytes in suspension with 10 μmol/l [^{14}C]GCDC in the presence or absence of 20 μmol/l ursodeoxycholate. After 30 min, 1 ml of the cell suspension was placed in microfuge tubes containing 200 μl of an oil mixture (one part bis(3,5,5-trimethylhexyl)phthalate to four parts bibutyl phthalate), and centrifuged for 30 s in a Beckman microfuge (model E, Beckman Instruments Inc., Palo Alto, CA). The pellet was resuspended in 1 ml of NCS solubilizing solution (0.9 ml of NCS tissue solubilizer plus 0.1 ml of water per vial). Pellets were heated at 60°C for 90 min, after which 30 ml of glacial acetic acid was added. The solubilized pellets were transferred to 8 ml of Optifluor (Packard Instrument Company Inc., CT).

Radioactivity was quantitated using a scintillation counter (Beckman model LS 6000 SC, Beckman Instruments Inc, Fullerton, CA).

Materials

Ursodeoxycholic acid and glycoursodeoxycholic acid were obtained from Calbiochem Corp (La Jolla, CA). [^{14}C]GCDC was obtained from Dr Alan F. Hoffman, UCSD, La Jolla, CA. All other bile salts and chemicals were obtained from Sigma Chemical Co. (St Louis, MO). The bile salts used were > 96% pure by thin-layer chromatography performed by the manufacturers, and were used without further purification.

RESULTS/DISCUSSION

Bile salt-induced hepatocyte apoptosis

We initially demonstrated by electron microscopy that the bile salt glycodeoxycholate (GDC) caused the characteristic ultrastructural morphological changes of apoptosis[15]. Furthermore, the typical inter-nucleosomal pattern of DNA cleavage was also observed in bile-salt-treated cells, but not in controls[15]. Both the morphological and biochemical features of GDC-induced apoptosis were inhibited by zinc sulphate (500 μmol/l), an endonuclease inhibitor. *In-vitro* studies of hepatocyte nuclear protein extract revealed that nuclear endonucleases were constitutively expressed and could be activated by Mg^{2+} in the absence of Ca^{2+}. Indeed, cytosolic free calcium did not change during incubation with GDC, although cytosolic free magnesium increased to twice basal values[15]. Based on these findings we postulate that GDC-induced apoptosis is promoted by an influx of Mg^{2+} into the cell, stimulating activity of Mg^{2+}-dependent endonucleases (Fig. 1).

These findings demonstrated for the first time that bile salts can cause hepatocyte injury by apoptosis. The extent of apoptosis was determined by incubating hepatocytes in culture media containing the bile salt of interest and quantitating the number of cells with nuclear fragmentation. Following exposure of hepatocytes to 50 μmol/l bile salt for 4 h, nuclear fragmentation was observed in 55 ± 2% of cells treated with GDC and 61 ± 10% of cells treated with glycochenodeoxycholate (GCDC), but not in controls.

We have previously demonstrated that toxic bile salts such as the deoxycholates and chenodeoxycholates can cause hepatocyte necrosis at concentrations of 250 μmol/l or greater[10]. The concentration of the toxic bile salt (e.g. GDC or GCDC) therefore determines whether a cell undergoes necrosis or apoptosis. Consequently, the type of hepatocellular injury during cholestasis may reflect the concentration of bile salt retained within the hepatocyte. Furthermore, the subcellular events occurring during bile salt toxicity must also be concentration-dependent. Indeed, bile-salt-induced apoptosis is characterized by maintenance of cellular ATP and structural integrity of mitochondria (data not shown) while GCDC-induced cell necrosis results in ATP depletion, inhibition of mitochondrial respiration and induction of the mitochondrial membrane permeability transition[17]. Thus the active, ATP-requiring process of apoptosis

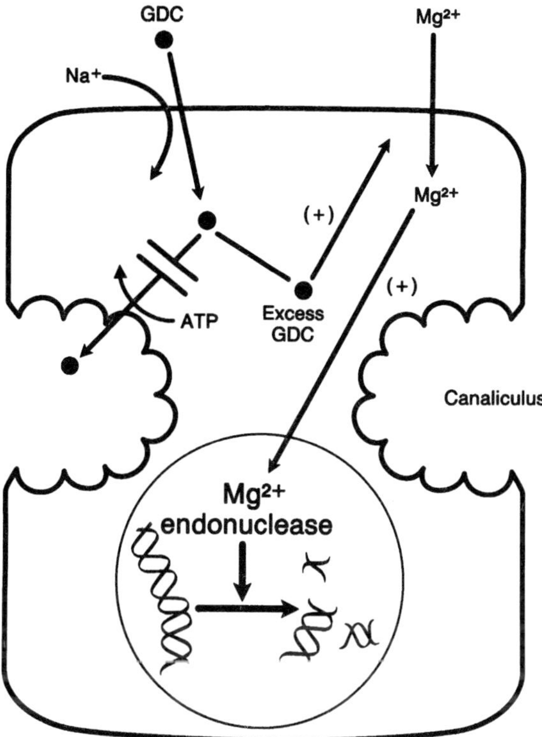

Fig. 1 Postulated sequence of intracellular events during bile-salt-induced hepatocyte apoptosis. During Cholestasis the retention of bile salts leads to an increased intracellular concentration of toxic bile salts such as GDC. An excess of intracellular GDC promotes an influx of magnesium, and elevation of intracellular magnesium, which enhances endogenous endonuclease activity

appears to occur when bile salt concentrations are insufficient to cause mitochondrial injury, whereas cell necrosis results when bile salt concentrations are sufficient to cause mitochondrial injury. Further work will be required to determine the specific role of mitochondria in bile salt-induced toxicity.

Relationship between bile salt hydrophobicity and toxicity

Bile salt hydrophobicity is a function of its structure and predictive of the biological and physicochemical properties of individual bile salts[18]. In addition, the hydrophobicity of bile salts has been reported to correlate with hepatotoxicity. To determine the relationship between bile salt hydrophobicity (hence structure) and toxicity, we evaluated both apoptosis and necrosis by a variety of bile salts. Published data were used for bile salt hydrophobicity[18]. Cell apoptosis was induced by incubating cells with 100 μmol/l bile salt for 4 h and morphologically determined by identifying nuclear fragmentation using fluorescence microscopy. Cell necrosis was induced in hepatocytes in suspension by using

250 μmol/l bile salt and fluorometrically determined using propidium iodide. Cell necrosis correlated with the extent of hydrophobicity, with relatively hydrophilic bile salts exhibiting little toxicity. Relatively hydrophobic bile acids (chenodeoxycholate, deoxycholate, lithocholate) were toxic in order of increasing hydrophobicity, with the exception of glycochenodeoxycholate, which was more toxic than any of the other bile salts studied (Fig. 2). These studies confirmed current concepts suggesting that hepatocyte necrosis was related to the hydrophobicity of bile salts[12,19]. In contrast, no relationship was observed between bile salt hydrophobicity and cell apoptosis (Fig. 3). These findings suggest that the tendency to induce apoptosis is unrelated to the structure and physicochemical properties of the individual bile salts. Furthermore, alterations in the plasma membrane or the release of membrane phospholipids is unlikely to be related to subsequent induction of apoptosis by bile salts.

Ursodeoxycholate and its conjugates inhibit GCDC-induced hepatocyte apoptosis

Exogenous administration of the bile salt ursodeoxycholate (UDC) ameliorates liver injury during cholestasis. However, the cellular mechanisms responsible

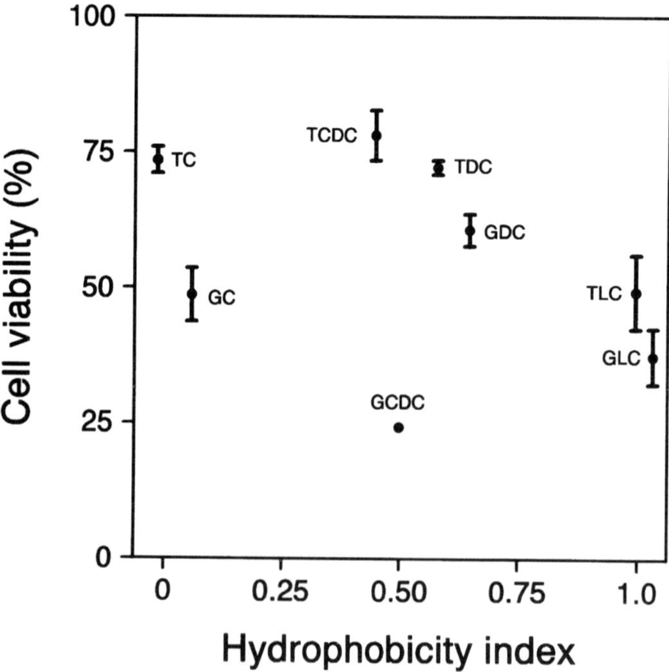

Fig. 2 Relationship between hydrophobicity and bile-salt-induced necrosis. Hepatocyte suspensions (10^5/ml) were incubated for 2 h with 250 μmol/l bile salt in 3 ml of KRH buffer containing 1 μmol/l propidium iodide and 0.2% BSA at 37°C. Cell necrosis and loss of viability was assessed by propidium iodide fluorometry. Cell viability after 2 h is plotted against bile salt hydrophobicity

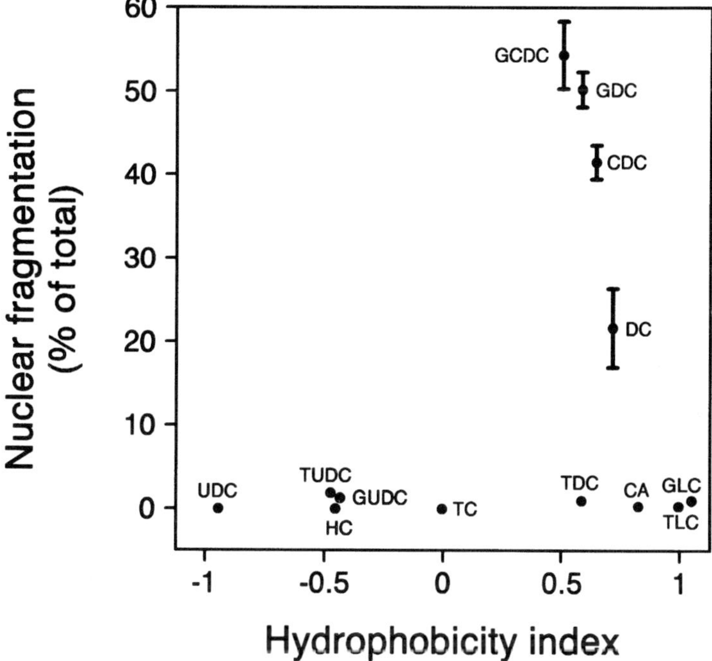

Fig. 3 Relationship between hydrophobicity and bile-salt-induced apoptosis. Cultured rat hepatocytes were incubated in culture media at 37°C with 100 μmol/l bile salt for 4 h. Cells were stained with 5 μmol/l acridine orange, transferred to a glass slide and viewed with a fluorescence microscope. At least 300 cells were counted. Nuclear fragmentation represents cells with at least three nuclear fragments expressed as a percentage of total cell counted

for cytoprotection by UDC remain poorly understood. UDC is absorbed and conjugated to glycine and taurine in the liver, and these conjugates are believed to displace toxic bile salts from the liver[20]. UDC protects against hepatocyte apoptosis during incubation with 50 μmol/l GCDC. Nuclear fragmentation was reduced 1.7-fold in the presence of 100 μmol/l UDC plus 50 μmol/l GCDC compared to cells incubated with GCDC alone (28.1 ± 5.1 vs. 48.9 ± 5.4% after 3 h incubation, $p<0.01$) (Fig. 4). Uptake studies were performed using [14C]GCDC and unlabelled UDC. Intracellular accumulation of [14C]GCDC was not significantly altered by the presence or absence of a 2-fold excess of UDC (1.07 ± 0.02 pmol/10^6 cells vs. 1.13 ± 0.01 pmol/10^6 cells). Thus, the protective effect of UDC was not due to a physicochemical interaction between UDC and GCDC in the incubation medium or at the hepatocyte plasma membrane preventing uptake of GCDC into hepatocytes. Furthermore, both taurine and glycine conjugates of UDC had a protective effect on GCDC-induced hepatocyte apoptosis. GCDC (50 μmol/l)-induced nuclear fragmentation was reduced by 65.6 ± 8.7% in the presence of 100 μmol/l tauroursodeoxycholate (TUDC) and by 79.4 ± 5.4% in the presence of 100 μmol/l glycoursodeoxycholate (GUDC) after 3 h (Fig. 4). These results indicate that the hepatoprotective effect

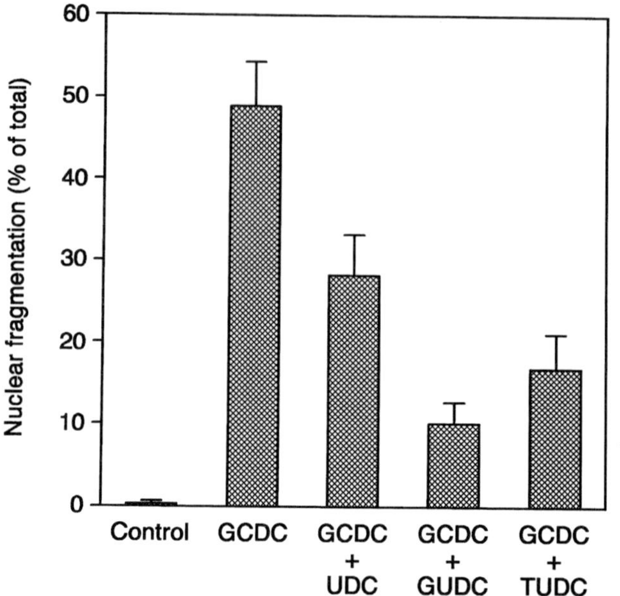

Fig. 4 Ursodeoxycholate and its conjugates inhibit GCDC-induced apoptosis. Cultured rat hepato-cytes were incubated in culture media at 37°C with 50 μmol/l GCDC for 4 h in the presence or absence of UDC, TUDC or GUDC. Cells were stained with 5 μmol/l acridine orange, transferred to a glass slide and viewed with a fluorescence microscope. At least 300 cells were counted. Nuclear fragmentation represents cells with at least three nuclear fragments expressed as a percentage of total cells counted

of UDC and its conjugates is far more complex than simple inhibition of toxic bile salt uptake by hepatocytes, and suggest an intracellular cytoprotective mechanism.

The criteria for cell injury currently used in the study of bile salt toxicity, such as the release of cellular enzymes (lactate deydrogenase, aminotrans-ferases) and the exclusion of trypan blue, detect the occurrence of cellular necro-sis but not apoptosis. Release of intracellular constituents and loss of plasma membrane integrity are not features of apoptotic cell death *in vivo*. Thus future studies of the mechanisms of bile salt hepatotoxicity and the effects of cytopro-tective agents such as UDC will need also to incorporate measures of cellular apoptosis.

Our studies demonstrate that toxic bile salts can cause hepatocellular injury by apoptosis as well as by cell necrosis. The common histopathological findings of sequelae of apoptosis (e.g. acidophilic bodies) in chronic cholestasis underscores the importance of bile-salt-induced apoptosis as a mechanism of hepatotoxicity in cholestatic liver disease. Elucidation of the mechanistic steps involved during bile-salt-induced hepatocyte apoptosis may provide targets for therapeutic interventions to ameliorate bile-salt-induced cytotoxicity.

Acknowledgements

This work was supported by the Mayo Foundation, Grant DK 41876 from the National Institutes of Health, the Gainey Foundation (G.J.G.), and by a AGA Foundation/Merck Senior Research Fellow award (T.P.).

References

1. Greim H, Trulzsch D, Roboz J *et al*. Mechanism of cholestasis. 5. Bile acids in normal rat livers and in those after bile duct ligation. Gastroenterology. 1972;63:837–45.
2. Greim H, Trulzsch D, Gzygan P *et al*. Mechanism of cholestasis. 6. Bile acids in human livers with or without biliary obstruction. Gastroenterology. 1972;62:846–50.
3. Heuman DM, Mills AS, McCall JB, Hylemon PB, Pandak WM, Vlahcevic ZR. Conjugates of ursodeoxycholate protect against cholestasis and hepatocellular necrosis caused by more hydrophobic bile salts: *in vivo* studies in the rat. Gastroenterology. 1991;100:203–11.
4. Gerschenson LE, Rotello RJ. Apoptosis: a different type of cell death. FASEB J. 1992;6:2450–5.
5. Rosser B, Gores G. Liver cell necrosis: cellular mechanisms and clinical implications. Gastroenterology. 1995;108:252–75.
6. Schwartzman R, Cidlowski J. Apoptosis: the biochemistry and molecular biology of programmed cell death. Endocr Rev. 1993;14:133–51.
7. Compton MA. A biochemical hallmark of apoptosis: internucleosomal degradation of the genome. Cancer Metast Rev. 1992;11:105–19.
8. Kerr JF, Wyllie AH, Currie AR. Apoptosis: a basic biological phenomenon with wideranging implications in tissue kinetics. Br J Cancer. 1972;26:239–57.
9. Zimniak P, Little JM, Radominska A, Oelberg DG, Anwer MS, Lester R. Taurine-conjugated bile acids act as calcium ionophores. Biochemistry. 1991;30:8598–604.
10. Spivey J, Bronk S, Gores G. Glycochenodeoxycholate-induced lethal hepatocellular injury in rat hepatocytes. Role of ATP depletion and cytosolic free calcium. J Clin Invest. 1993;92:17–24.
11. Billington D, Evans CE, Godfrey PP, Coleman R. Effects of bile acids on the plasma membranes of isolated rat hepatocytes. Biochem J. 1980;88:321 7.
12. Attili AF, Angelico M, Cantafora A, Alvaro D, Capocaccia L. Bile acid-induced liver toxicity: relation to the hydrophobic-hydrophilic balance of bile acids. Med Hypoth. 1986;19:57–69.
13. Anwer MS, Engelking LR, Nolan K, Sullivan D, Zimniak P, Lester R. Hepatotoxic bile acids increase cytosolic calcium activity of isolated rat hepatocytes. Hepatology. 1991;8:887–91.
14. Searle J, Harmon BV, Bishop CJ, Kerr JFR. The significance of cell death by apoptosis in hepatobiliary disease. J Gastro Hepatol. 1987;2:77–96.
15. Patel T, Bronk S, Gores G. Increases of intracellular magnesium promote glycodeoxycholate-induced apoptosis in rat hepatocytes. J Clin Invest. 1994;94:2183–92.
16. Gores GJ, Nieminen A-L, Fleishman KE, Dawson TL, Herman B, Lemasters JJ. Extracellular acidosis delays onset of cell death in ATP-depleted hepatocytes. Am J Physiol. 1988;255(Cell Physiol. 24):C315–22.
17. Spivey J, Botla R, Bronk S, Gores G. The hydrophobic bile salt as an agent of mitochondrial toxicity. In: Bile acids in gastroenterology: basic and clinical advances. Lancaster; Kluwer; 1995 (In press)
18. Heuman D. Quantitative estimation of the hydrophilic–hydrophobic balance of mixed bile salt solutions. J Lipid Res. 1989;30:719–30.
19. Scholmerich J, Becher M, Schmidt K, Schubert R, Kremer B. Influence of hydroxylation and conjugation of bile salts on their membrane damaging properties – studies on isolated hepatocytes and lipid membrane vesicles. Hepatology. 1984;4:661–6.
20. Ohiwa T, Katagiri K, Hoshino M, Hayakawa T, Nakai T. Tauroursodeoxycholate and tauro-β-muricholate exert cytoprotection by reducing intrahepatic taurochenodeoxycholate content. Hepatology. 1993;17:470–6.

10
Bile acids and hepatocellular signalling

U. BEUERS, G.-A. KULLAK-UBLICK and G. PAUMGARTNER

Numerous functions of the liver cell, such as bile secretion, carbohydrate, lipid and protein synthesis and degradation, or biotransformation, are regulated by a network of intracellular and transmembraneous signalling mechanisms which are at present incompletely elucidated. In recent years the important role of messenger systems in the control of hepatocellular functions has been increasingly recognized[1].

Bile acids have long been known to act as the primary osmotic driving force for bile formation[2]. Physicochemical properties of numerous bile acid species have been characterized[3], and the transport kinetics of bile acids across the hepatocyte have been studied intensely[4–6]. It has only recently been suggested, however, that bile acids may affect liver cell functions by modulating hepatocellular signalling mechanisms. The aim of this chapter is to present a brief overview of studies investigating the effect of bile acids on hepatocellular signalling mechanisms.

Cytosolic free calcium $[Ca^{2+}]_i$ plays a critical role in the control of many hepatocellular functions including bile secretion[7]. Anwer *et al.*[8] and Combettes *et al.*[9–11] were the first to show that hydrophobic bile acids such as taurolithocholic acid (TLCA) or taurochenodeoxycholic acid (TCDCA), but not taurocholic acid (TCA) at high micromolar concentrations affect $[Ca^{2+}]_i$ in isolated rat hepatocytes. The increase in $[Ca^{2+}]_i$ was shown to be due to depletion of endoplasmic inositol 1,4,5-trisphosphate (IP_3)-sensitive Ca^{2+} stores independent of the formation of IP_3. It was controversially discussed whether Ca^{2+} influx across the plasma membrane contributed to TLCA-induced $[Ca^{2+}]_i$ increase in the liver cell[8–11]. In addition, it was demonstrated that hydrophobic bile acids such as TLCA, TCDCA or taurodeoxycholic acid (TDCA), but not hydrophobic bile acids such as TCA or tauroursodeoxycholic acid (TUDCA) induced Ca^{2+} efflux from isolated hepatocytes at high micromolar concentrations[12]. In contrast, biliary Ca^{2+} secretion was markedly stimulated by GUDCA, but not by TCDCA in the perfused rat liver[13]. On the basis of these experimental findings it was speculated[8,9] that (T)LCA-induced liver cell damage and cholestasis might be mediated by (T)LCA-induced changes in hepatocellular $[Ca^{2+}]_i$.

Using the perfused rat liver, Farrell and co-workers[14] presented experimental evidence that release of Ca^{2+} from the endoplasmic reticulum is not the mechanism for bile acid-induced cholestasis and hepatotoxicity. Their experiments were supported by the finding that the hydrophilic non-toxic bile acid tauroursodeoxycholic acid (TUDCA) was a more potent Ca^{2+} agonist in neutrophils[15] as well as in hepatocytes[16] than its hydrophobic epimer TCDCA. First reports on the beneficial effect of the hydrophilic bile acid ursodeoxycholic acid (UDCA) in the treatment of chronic cholestasis liver disease[17–20] created interest in the effect of UDCA and its conjugates on cellular signalling mechanisms[15,16,21] including $[Ca^{2+}]_i$. In isolated rat hepatocytes in short-term culture, TUDCA caused a sustained increase in $[Ca^{2+}]_i$ at concentrations as low as 1 μmol/l, reaching a maximum effect at 5 μmol/l, which is within the physiological range of serum bile acid levels[16]. The sustained $[Ca^{2+}]_i$ increase induced by 10 μmol/l TUDCA was significantly higher than that induced by any other bile acid tested at equimolar concentrations under identical experimental conditions[16]. The (T)UDCA-induced increase in $[Ca^{2+}]_i$ was due to: (a) depletion of IP_3-sensitive endoplasmic Ca^{2+} stores independent of IP_3 (thus, independent of the activation of phospholipase C)[16,21], and (b) stimulation of Ca^{2+} influx across the plasma membrane[16,21,22] via Ni^{2+}-sensitive Ca^{2+} channels[22].

A sustained increase of $[Ca^{2+}]_i$ is the key signal for the stimulation of exocytosis in a number of secretory cells by molecular mechanisms which are at present unknown (for review see ref. 23). In hepatocytes, biliary exocytosis (i.e. vesicle fusion with the canalicular membrane) may be of dual importance: (a) secretion of high molecular weight proteins and lipophilic anions including bile acids[24], and (b) targeting and insertion of transport proteins into the canalicular membrane (possibly more important for the maintenance of the transport function of the liver cell)[25]. Studies in the perfused rat liver using horseradish peroxidase (HRP) as an established marker of the vesicular pathway in hepatocytes revealed that TUDCA, but not the primary bile acids TCA and TCDCA at physiological portovenous concentrations, induced a marked and sustained stimulation of biliary exocytosis[22]. This effect of TUDCA was dependent on the mobilization of extracellular Ca^{2+} by the hepatocytes[22].

Biliary exocytosis and bile secretory capacity of the liver cell are impaired in experimental cholestasis[22]. In cholestatic hepatocytes of bile duct-ligated animals, Ca^{2+} influx across the plasma membrane via Ni^{2+}-sensitive Ca channels is also impaired[22], suggesting a potential connection. In line with these findings, Berridge and co-workers reported experiments in the perfused rat liver indicating that transmembraneous Ca^{2+} fluxes are impaired in different experimental models of cholestasis[26].

These data could be an indication that UDCA exerts its beneficial effect in cholestatic liver disease in part by stimulating vesicle fusion and insertion of transport proteins into the canalicular membrane of the hepatocyte in a Ca^{2+}-dependent way[22].

Häussinger *et al.* reported that TUDCA at low micromolar concentrations induces cell swelling of hepatocytes and stimulates TCA secretion into bile[27]. Interestingly, the V_{max} of biliary TCA secretion was increased by TUDCA in this study, suggesting that the canalicular transport capacity for TCA, i.e. the number of functionally active bile acid transport proteins inserted into the canalicular membrane, was enhanced by TUDCA at low micromolar concentrations[27]. It would be interesting to know whether TUDCA-induced cell swelling in the hepatocyte is mediated by $[Ca^{2+}]_i$. A comparison of the effect of TUDCA with those of more hydrophobic bile acids such as TCDCA on cell swelling could help to assess whether TUDCA-induced cell swelling may contribute to the beneficial effect of UDCA in cholestasis liver disease.

In addition to the effect of TUDCA on secretory mechanisms, (T)UDCA-induced modulation of carbohydrate metabolism was demonstrated in isolated hepatocytes: glycogen phosphorylase a was stimulated by UDCA[21] and glucose release of isolated hepatocytes in short-term culture was stimulated by TUDCA[16], both Ca^{2+}-dependent mechanisms. In contrast, an effect of TUDCA on glucose release was not observed in the perfused rat liver[13] (K. Jungermann, personal communication). This difference remains unexplained.

It is tempting to speculate that the effect of TUDCA on $[Ca^{2+}]_i$ may also affect other mechanisms involved in hepatocellular secretion. Canalicular contractions have been shown[28] to be modulated by changes in $[Ca^{2+}]_i$, and preliminary studies in hepatocyte couplets provided evidence for TUDCA-induced stimulation of canalicular contractions[29]. Whether TUDCA-induced changes in $[Ca^{2+}]_i$ may modulate the permeability of the tight junctions, as has been reported for the Ca^{2+} agonist vasopressin[30], is at present unclear. Further studies are necessary to elucidate the molecular mechanisms involved in TUDCA-induced stimulation of regulated exocytosis.

In addition of $[Ca^{2+}]_i$, the protein kinase C family of isoenzymes (PKC) and cyclic AMP-dependent protein kinase A (PKA) are intracellular modulators of bile flow and exocytosis in hepatocytes[1]. Experimental evidence indicates that exocytosis is stimulated by activation of PKA[31], as well as PKC[32], although the exact molecular mechanisms remain unclear. Bouscarel *et al.*[33] have provided experimental evidence indicating that UDCA does not affect basal levels of cAMP in hepatocytes, although glucagon-induced increase of hepatocellular cAMP levels were reduced by UDCA[33]. This indicates that the basal activity of PKA is not markedly affected by UDCA.

It is generally accepted that the activation of PKC involves two steps: (a) translocation of the enzyme from cytosol to the membranes and (b) binding of the intracellular activator diacylglycerol to the enzyme[34,35]. In hepatocytes the Ca^{2+}-dependent conventional isoforms α and (probably) ß, as well as the Ca^{2+}-independent isoforms δ, ϵ, and ζ are expressed, as determined by Western blotting[36,37]. In isolated hepatocytes, TUDCA (10 μmol/l) induced translocation of the α-isoform, but not δ-, ϵ- and ζ-PKC, whereas TCA at equimolar concentrations did not affect distribution of PKC isoform in hepatocytes[36]. UDCA (100 μmol/l) was also shown to induce translocation of conventional PKC (using a/β monoclonal anti-PKC antibody) and to stimulate phosphorylation of a 80 kDa protein, a substrate of PKC[33]. In addition, TUDCA (10 μmol/l) and TCA (10 μmol/l) significantly increased diacylglycerol mass in isolated hepatocytes[38]. These data suggest that (T)UDCA activates α-PKC in isolated hepatocytes. This isoform is of specific interest with regard to regulation of exocytosis because α-PKC has been demonstrated to mediate opening of membrane Ca^{2+}-channels and stimulation of exocytosis in different cell types[39,40].

In summary, a number of studies performed during recent years indicate that bile acids may act as potent hepatocellular signalling agonists. Modulation of signalling pathways may depend on the structure and physicochemical properties of a bile acid, as demonstrated by the variability of the effects induced by different bile acids on $[Ca^{2+}]_i$. The exact molecular mechanisms by which bile acids modulate signalling mechanisms in the liver cell remain to be determined. However, it is interesting that bile acids at physiological concentrations may modulate hepatocellular functions by potently interacting with a complex hepatocellular signal network.

References

1. Nathanson M, Boyer JL. Mechanisms and regulation of bile secretion. Hepatology. 1991;14:551–66.
2. Boyer JL. New concepts of mechanisms of hepatocyte bile formation. Physiol Rev. 1980;60:303–26.
3. Hofmann AF, Schteingart CD, Hagey LR. Species differences in bile acid metabolism. In: Paumgartner G, Beuers U, editors. Bile acids in liver diseases. Lancaster: Kluwer; 1995:3–30.
4. Hagenbuch B, Stieger B, Meier P. Hepatocellular basolateral bile acid uptake. In: Paumgartner G, Beuers U, editors. Bile acids in liver diseases. Lancaster: Kluwer; 1995:49–55.
5. Crawford JM. Transcellular bile acid transport. In: Paumgartner G, Beuers U, editors. Bile acids in liver diseases. Lancaster: Kluwer; 1995:56–62.
6. Keppler D, Mayer R, Böhme M, Büchler M. Bile acid transport across the canalicular membrane. In: Paumgartner G, Beuers U, editors. Bile acids in liver diseases. Lancaster: Kluwer; 1995:63–67.
7. Exton JH. Role of phosphoinositides in the regulation of liver function. Hepatology. 1989;8:152–66.
8. Anwer MS, Engelking LR, Sullivan D, Zimniak P, Lester R. Hepatotoxic bile acids increase cytosolic Ca^{++} activity of isolated rat hepatocytes. Hepatology. 1988;8:887–91.
9. Combettes L, Dumont M, Berthon B, Erlinger S, Claret M. Release of calcium from the endoplasmic reticulum by bile acids in rat liver cells. J Biol Chem. 1988;263:2299–303.
10. Combettes L, Berthon B, Doucet E, Erlinger S, Claret M. Characteristics of bile acid-mediated Ca^{++} release from permeabilized liver cells and liver microsomes. J Biol Chem. 1989;264:157–67.
11. Combettes L, Berthon B, Doucet E, Erlinger S, Claret M. Bile acids mobilise internal Ca^{++} independently of external Ca^{++} in rat hepatocytes. Eur J Biochem. 1990;190:619–23.
12. Anwer MS, Little JM, Oelberg DG, Zimniak P, Lester R. Effect of bile acids on Ca^{++} efflux from isolated rat hepatocytes and perfused rat livers. Proc Soc Exp Biol Med. 1989;191:147–52.
13. Hamada Y, Karjalainen A, Setchell BA, Millard JE. Acute effects of cholestatic and choleretic bile salts on vasopressin- and glucagon-induced hepato-biliary calcium fluxes in the perfused rat liver. Biochem J. 1992;283:575–81.
14. Farrell GC, Duddy SK, Kass GEN, Llopis J, Gahm A, Orrenius S. Release of Ca^{++} from the endoplasmic reticulum is not the mechanism for bile acid-induced cholestasis and hepatotoxicity in the intact liver. J Clin Invest. 1990;85:1255–9.
15. Beuers U, Thiel M, Bardenheuer H, Paumgartner G. Tauroursodeoxycholic acid inhibits the cytosolic Ca^{++} increase in human neutrophils stimulated by formyl-methionyl-leucyl-phenylalanine. Biochem Biophys Res Commun. 1990;171:1115–21.
16. Beuers U, Nathanson MH, Boyer JL. Effects of tauroursodeoxycholic acid on cytosolic Ca^{++} signals in isolated rat hepatocytes. Gastroenterology. 1993;104:604–12.
17. Poupon R, Poupon RE, Calmus, Y, Ballet F, Darnis F. Is ursodeoxycholic acid an effective treatment for primary biliary cirrhosis? Lancet. 1987;1:834–6.
18. Leuschner U, Fischer H, Kurtz W *et al.* Ursodeoxycholic acid in primary biliary cirrhosis: results of a controlled double-blind trial. Gastroenterology. 1989;97:1268–74.
19. Poupon RE, Balkau B, Eschwege E, Poupon R, and the UDCA–PBC study group. A multicenter, controlled trial of ursodiol for the treatment of primary biliary cirrhosis. N Engl J Med 1991;324:1548–54.

20. Beuers U, Spengler U, Kruis W *et al*. Ursodeoxycholic acid for treatment of primary sclerosing cholangitis. Hepatology. 1992;16:707–14.
21. Bouscarel B, Fromm H, Nussbaum R. Ursodeoxycholate mobilizes intracellular Ca^{++} and activates phosphorylase *a* in isolated hepatocytes. Am J Physiol. 1993;264:G243–51.
22. Beuers U, Nathanson MH, Isales CM, Boyer JL. Tauroursodeoxycholic acid stimulates hepatocellular exocytosis and mobilizes extracellular Ca^{++}, mechanisms defective in cholestasis. J Clin Invest. 1993;92:2984–93.
23. Burgoyne RD, Morgan A. Regulated exocytosis. Biochem J. 1993;293:305–16.
24. Crawford JM, Gollan JL. Transcellular transport of organic anions: still a long way to go. Hepatology. 1991;14:192–7.
25. Boyer JL, Roelofsen H, Soroka CJ. Vesicle targeting to the canalicular domain regulates bile acid transport and bile secretory function in the liver. In: Paumgartner G, Beuers U, editors. Bile acids in liver diseases. Lancaster: Kluwer; 1995:109–112.
26. Hamada Y, Karjalainen A, Bygrave FL. Hormone – induced bile flow and hepatobiliary calcium fluxes are attenuated in the perfused liver of rats made cholestatic with ethynylestradiol in vivo and with phalloidin in vitro. Hepatology. 1995;21:1455–64.
27. Häussinger D, Hallbrucker C, Saha N, Lang F. Cell volume and bile acid excretion. Biochem J. 1992;288:681–9.
28. Watanabe S, Tomono M, Takeuchi M *et al*. Bile canalicular contraction in the isolated hepatocyte doublet is related to an increase in cytosolic free calcium ion concentration. Liver. 1988;8:178–83.
29. Oda M, Kazemoto S, Kaneko H *et al*. Involvement of pericanalicular ectoplasmic free calcium ion and Ca^{++}-Mg^{++}-ATPase in the bile acid-induced enhancement and impairment of bile canalicular contractions Hepatology. 1992;16:118A (abstract).
30. Nathanson MH, Gautam A, Ng OC, Bruck R, Boyer JL. Hormonal regulation of paracellular permeability in isolated rat hepatocyte couplets. Am J Physiol. 1992;262:G1079–86.
31. Benedetti A, Strazzabosco M, Ng OC, Boyer JL. Regulation of activity and apical targeting of the Cl⁻/HCO3⁻ exchanger in rat hepatocytes. Proc Natl Acad Sci USA. 1994;91:792–6.
32. Bruck R, Nathanson MH, Roelofsen H, Boyer JL. Effects of protein kinase C and cytosolic Ca^{++} on exocytosis in the isolated perfused rat liver. Hepatology. 1994;20:1032–40.
33. Bouscarel B, Grettys TW, Fromm H, Dubner H. Ursodeoxycholic acid inhibits glucagon-induced cAMP formation in hamster hepatocytes: a role for PKC. Am J Physiol. 1995;268:G300–10.
34. Nishizuka Y. Intracellular signalling by hydrolysis of phospholipids and activation of protein kinase C. Science. 1992;258:607–14.
35. Hug H, Sarre TF. Protein kinase C isoenzymes: divergence in signal transduction? Biochem J. 1993;291:329–43.
36. Beuers U, Throckmorton DO, Anderson MH, Isales CM, Boyer JL. Tauroursodeoxycholic acid induces translocation of α-, but not δ-, ϵ-, and ζ-protein kinase C in rat hepatocytes. Hepatology. 1993;18:135A (abstract).
37. Kosaka Y, Ogita K, Ase K, Nomura H, Kikkawa U, Nishizuka Y. The hererogeneity of protein kinase C in various rat tissues. Biochem Biophys Res Commun. 1988;151:973–81.
38. Beuers U, Sauter G, Koebe HG, Paumgartner G. Tauroursodeoxycholic acid stimulates formation of sn-1,2-diacylglycerol in isolated rat hepatocytes. Gastroenterology. 1995;108:1035A (abstract).
39. Riedel H, Parissenti AM, Hansen H, Su L, Shieh HL. Stimulation of Ca uptake in *Saccharomyces cerevisiae* by bovine protein kinase C a. J Biol Chem. 1993;268:3456–62.
40. Ganesan S, Calle R, Zawalich K, Smallwood JI, Zawalich WS, Rasmussen H. Glucose-induced translocation of protein kinase C in rat pancreatic islets. Proc Natl Acad Sci USA. 1990;87:9893–7.

11
Hepatobiliary cholesterol secretion and the function of mdr2 P-glycoprotein

R. P. J. OUDE ELFERINK, C. FRIJTERS, R. OTTENHOFF,
M. VAN WIJLAND and A. K. GROEN

mdr2 P-GLYCOPROTEIN AS A PHOSPHATIDYLCHOLINE TRANSLOCATOR

Bile formation is critically dependent on a number of ATP-dependent transport functions in the canalicular plasma membrane. Bile salts are pumped against a high concentration gradient into the canalicular lumen. By an as-yet-unknown mechanism luminal bile salts catalyse the secretion of phospholipid and cholesterol. Until recently it was assumed that the latter process is passively mediated by the detergent action of bile salt on the canalicular membrane.

The production of a knockout mouse for mdr2 P-glycoprotein (Pgp) has, however, demonstrated that this process requires the function of this canalicular membrane protein[1]. P-glycoprotein represent a small family of isozymes. In mice three genes encode for Pgps: *mdr1a*, *mdr1b* and *mdr2*. In humans two genes were characterized, *MDR1* and *MDR3*. High homology was observed between the mouse *mdr2* and the human *MDR3* genes. Analysis of the genes revealed that they encoded for so-called ABC transporters; a large family of proteins which possess ATP-binding domains and are involved in active transmembrane transport[2,3]. Overexpression of *mdr1a* and *mdr1b* Pgp renders cells resistant towards amphipathic cytotoxic drugs[4,5]. It was demonstrated that they function in the extrusion of these drugs from the cells, thereby keeping the intracellular concentration low. This could not be demonstrated for mdr2 Pgp; therefore this protein must have another function. The expression of the various Pgps in normal tissues is also quite different; the mouse mdr2 Pgp and human MDR3 Pgp are predominantly expressed in the canalicular membrane of the hepatocyte, and to a lesser extent also in muscle and spleen[6-8].

It was observed that mice in which the gene for mdr2 Pgp was disrupted do not secrete phospholipid into bile[1]. In addition a very strong decrease in cholesterol secretion was found. Thus, bile from *mdr2* knockout mice is almost devoid of lipids while bile salt secretion is normal. Glutathione secretion is also severely decreased. Fortunately, it could be readily inferred which of these changes represented the primary defect: heterozygotes for *mdr2* gene disruption, which have about 50% of the normal expression had a normal bile composition except for a 40% decrease in phospholipid content. This strongly suggested that mdr2 Pgp is primarily involved in the biliary secretion of phospholipids. Based on its homology with the other Pgps it was hypothesized that mdr2 Pgp is also a transporter, and thus that it might function as a flippase which translocates phosphatidylcholine from the inner to the outer leaflet of the canalicular membrane[1].

Subsequent experiments with model systems in which mdr2 Pgp or its human homologue, MDR3 Pgp, were overexpressed supported this hypothesis. Ruetz and Gros[9] transfected the mouse *mdr2* gene in a yeast secretion mutant; at elevated temperature this mutant is unable to transport proteins to the plasma membrane, and as a consequence *de novo* synthesized plasma membrane proteins accumulate in intracellular secretory vesicles. These vesicles can be relatively easily harvested after homogenization of the cells, and they have the proper inside-out configuration for assaying transport from the cytoplasmic to the exoplasmic space. Using this experimental model the translocation of NBD-labelled phosphatidylcholine from the outer to the inner leaflet of the vesicles was determined. ATP-dependent translocation of NBD-PC was observed which was specific for mdr2 Pgp; it could not be observed in vesicles from yeast cells that were transfected with mdr1 or with the transfection vector alone. The fraction of PC molecules that was translocated was very low. This may, however, be expected, since the translocation process induces a phospholipid imbalance between the inner and outer leaflet, which is thermodynamically highly unfavourable. Thus, in the absence of net extraction of phospholipid from the *trans*-side of the bilayer, the translocation will halt. Unfortunately, little information was obtained on the substrate specificity of transport. It was not described whether the NBD moiety was present in the head group or in the fatty acid tail of the phosphosphatidylcholine molecule. Interestingly, the translocation could be inhibited by low concentrations of verapamil, which is an inhibitor of mdr1 Pgp. This suggests, unexpectedly, that verapamil is able to inhibit mdr1 as well as mdr2 Pgp.

Further evidence supporting the flippase function of mdr2 Pgp was provided by Smith *et al.*[10], who used fibroblasts from transgenic mice that express MDR3, the human homologue of mdr2 Pgp. After metabolic labelling of intracellular phosphatidylcholine with radioactive choline, translocation from the inner to the outer leaflet was assayed, and this was compared with normal mouse fibroblasts which do not express *mdr2*. Translocation of radioactive phosphatidylcholine to the outer leaflet was measured by the possibility to exchange with phosphatidylcholine-transfer protein and liposomes in the medium. In *MDR3* expressing fibroblasts a more rapid translocation of PC was observed than in control fibroblasts.

These two studies suggest that mdr2 Pgp is indeed an ATP-dependent phosphatidylcholine translocator. Berr *et al.*[11] had previously described a flippase activity in rat liver canalicular membranes. Similar to the classical studies of

Bishop and Bell[12], which described a flippase activity in the endoplasmic reticulum, they used radioactive dibutyroyl-PC as ligand for transport. Due to its short, four-carbon, fatty acid chains this compound is highly water-soluble. Considerable translocation activity was observed in canalicular membranes, which was even higher than in microsomal preparations, but this activity was ATP-independent. It is therefore unlikely that this activity represents mdr2 Pgp. Indeed, identical experiments were performed in our laboratory, using canalicular membranes from control and *mdr2* knockout mice and similar activities were observed (C. Frijters, unpublished observations).What this flippase activity represents is, as yet, unclear. First, it is important to mention that conventionally purified canalicular membrane preparations are contaminated with other intracellular membranes, notably endoplasmic reticulum. It is therefore not certain whether this activity represents a canalicular flippase. However, if it is a canalicular protein it probably does not play a role in biliary PC secretion unless its function is strictly dependent on mdr2 Pgp activity, since under all conditions phospholipid secretion is negligible in the *mdr2* knockout mouse (see below).

THE ROLE OF mdr2 P-GLYCOPROTEIN IN CHOLESTEROL SECRETION

The studies described above suggest that mdr2 Pgp indeed functions in the translocation of phosphatidylcholine from the inner to the outer leaflet of the canalicular membrane. Since mdr2 Pgp is a primary active, ATP-dependent transporter it may create a surplus of phospholipids in the outer leaflet of the plasma membrane. Since this is thermodynamically unfavourable, this process could lead to phospholipid vesiculation from the outer leaflet under the influence of luminal bile salts. In the absence of mdr2 Pgp (in the mdr2 knockout (–/–) mice) no phospholipid secretion is observed. Apparently the outer leaflet of the canalicular membrane is highly resistant towards bile salt micelles. But how does this hold for cholesterol? As described above, the endogenous secretion of cholesterol is severely decreased in the *mdr2* knockout mouse. This fits with the conventional thought that phospholipid and cholesterol are secreted as intact units. However, the endogenous bile salt pool of mice is very hydrophilic, consisting of about 70% of muricholate, with the remainder being taurocholate. When mdr2 (–/–) mice were infused with more hydrophobic bile salts such as taurocholate or taurodeoxycholate the phospholipid secretion remained low, but cholesterol secretion increased to substantial levels (Table 1). Thus, by changing the hydrophobicity of the secreted bile salts, we were able to partially uncouple cholesterol and phospholipid secretion. It could be argued that this is a consequence of the cytotoxic bile that is secreted. However, a similar, albeit lower, cholesterol secretion in the mdr2 (–/–) mice was observed when large quantities of the hydrophilic, non-toxic, bile salt tauroursodeoxycholate were infused. In order to exclude the increased cholesterol secretion being a consequence of the acute infusion of large amounts of bile salts, we fed control and *mdr2* knockout mice a diet to which 0.1% cholate was added. After 3 weeks the gallbladder was cannulated and bile was collected. Table 2 shows that, under these conditions also, an increased cholesterol secretion was observed in (–/–) mice fed with

Table 1 Biliary lipid secretion (nmol/min per 100 g) in control (+/+) and *mdr2* knockout (–/–) mice before and after infusion of taurodeoxycholate

	(+/+)	(–/–)
Endogenous secretion		
Bile salt	372 ± 116	454 ± 36 n.s.
Phospholipid	40 ± 13	0.65 ± 0.77***
Cholesterol	4.1 ± 1.5	n.d.***
Maximal secretion during infusion of taurodeoxycholate		
Bile salt	220 ± 19	169 ± 22*
Phospholipid	54 ± 6	1.1 ± 0.4***
Cholesterol	2.4 ± 0.2	2.1 ± 0.47**

Control (+/+) and *mdr2* knockout (–/–) mice were cannulated in the bile duct and bile was collected for 90 min. Subsequently, taurodeoxycholate was infused via the tail vein at a rate of 200 nmol/min and bile was collected for another 150 min. Values in the table represent the secretion of biliary components directly after cannulation (endogenous secretion) and during maximal secretion of taurodeoxycholate

cholate as compared with (–/–) mice on control diet. The table also shows that, although detectable, phospholipid secretion in (–/–) mice on cholate diet remains very low.

These data contradict the idea that phospholipid secretion and cholesterol secretion into bile are tightly coupled; in the absence of PC translocation the membrane is resistant towards bile salt-mediated phospholipid extraction; neither is there any vesicular secretion in this animal. Nevertheless cholesterol secretion does take place to a considerable extent, and this must take place by direct extraction from the membrane. The limited extent to which this occurs in (–/–) mice may be caused by the fact that the bile salt micelles in these animals do not contain phospholipids and therefore have a reduced affinity for cholesterol[13].

Table 2 Biliary lipid secretion (nmol/min per 100 g) in *mdr2* (+/+) and (–/–) mice on control diet and diet supplemented with 0.1% cholate

	(+/+)	(–/–)
Mice on control diet		
Bile salt	166 ± 83	297 ± 15 n.s.
Phospholipid	9.5 ± 3.3	n.d.***
Cholesterol	1.4 ± 0.5	n.d.***
Mice on 0.1% cholate		
Bile salt	433 ± 60	624 ± 98 n.s.
Phospholipid	77 ± 6	2.5 ± 01.3***
Cholesterol	15 ± 2	6.2 ± 0.7**

Mice were fed with a synthetic diet either, or not, supplemented with 0.1% cholate directly after weaning. After 3 weeks on this diet the animals were cannulated in the gallbladder and bile was collected. Bile that was obtained during the first 10 min after cannulation was assayed for the indicated component

The question now arises as to how cholesterol secretion takes place in normal mice. Two mechanisms could be envisaged. Either cholesterol could be directly extracted from the outer leaflet of the canalicular membrane, as occurs in the (–/–) animals, or cholesterol could laterally diffuse into the microdomains which are formed by mdr2 Pgp-mediated PC translocation and which (putatively) give rise to lipid vesicles; then cholesterol would be co-secreted with PC upon release of these vesicles. When these possibilities are considered it should be borne in mind that the phospholipid : cholesterol ratio in bile is quite different from that in the canalicular membrane. Although no direct data are available from the mouse, many studies in the rat have shown that the PC : cholesterol ratio in bile is about 10, while the value is between 1 and 2 in the canalicular membrane. If cholesterol is exclusively secreted via vesicles after lateral diffusion into microdomains, the amount of cholesterol secreted into bile will be critically dependent on the surface or the number of these domains, and thus on the activity of Pgp.

References

1. Smit JJM, Schinkel AH, Oude Elferink RPJ *et al.* Homozygous disruption of the murine mdr2 P-glycoprotein gene leads to a complete absence of phospholipid from bile and to liver disease. Cell. 1993;75:45–62.
2. Endicott JA, Ling V. The biochemistry of P-glycoprotein-mediated multidrug resistance. Annu Rev Biochem. 1989;58:137–71.
3. Gottesman MM, Pastan I. Biochemistry of multidrug resistance mediated by the multidrug transporter. Annu Rev Biochem. 1993,284.278–84.
4. Ueda K, Cardarelli C, Gottesman MM, Pastan I. Expression of a full-length cDNA for the human 'MDR1' gene confers resistance to colchicine, doxorubicin, and vinblastine. Proc Natl Acad Sci USA. 1987;84:3004–8.
5. Hammond JR, Johnstone RM, Gros P. Enhanced efflux of [3H] vinblastine from Chinese hamster ovary cells transfected with a full-length complementary DNA clone for the mdr1 gene. Cancer Res. 1989;49:3867–71.
6. van der Bliek AM, Baas F, ten Houte de Lange T *et al.* The human MDR3 gene encodes a novel P-glycoprotein homologue and gives rise to alternative spliced mRNAs in liver. EMBO J. 1987;6:3325–31.
7. Croop JM, Raymond M, Haber D *et al.* The three mouse multidrug resistance (mdr) genes are expressed in a tissue specific manner in normal mouse tissues. Mol Cell Biol. 1989;9:1346–50.
8. Buschman E, Arceci RJ, Croop JM *et al.* mdr2 encodes P-glycoprotein expressed in the bile canalicular membrane as determined by isoform-specific antibodies. J Biol Chem. 1992;267:18093–9.
9. Ruetz S, Gros P. Phosphatidylcholine translocase: a physiological role for the mdr2 gene. Cell. 1994;77:1071–82.
10. Smith AJ, Timmermans-Hereijgers JLPM, Roelofsen B *et al.* The human MDR3 P-glycoprotein promotes translocation of phosphatidylcholine through the plasma membrane of fibroblasts from transgenic mice. FEBS Lett. 1994;354:263–6.
11. Berr F, Meier PJ, Stieger B. Evidence for the presence of a phosphatidylcholine translocator in isolated rat liver canalicular plasma membrane vesicles. J Biol Chem. 1993;268:3976–9.
12. Bishop WR, Bell RM. Assembly of the endoplasmic reticulum phospholipid bilayer: the phosphatidylcholine transporter. Cell. 1985;42:51–60.
13. Carey MC, Small DM. The physical chemistry of cholesterol solubility in bile. Relationship to gallstone formation and dissolution in man. J Clin Invest. 1978;61:998–1026.

Section IV
Bile secretory function of liver and bile duct cells

12
Vesicle targeting to the canalicular domain regulates bile acid transport and bile secretory function in the liver

J. L. BOYER, H. ROELOFSEN and C. J. SOROKA

During the past two decades a large number of transport systems have been identified that are involved in the process of hepatic bile formation[1]. Many current studies are focusing on how some of these transporters may be regulated.

Regulation of membrane transport activity can occur through several different mechanisms: the turnover rate or half-life of the protein may be altered; the catalytic activity of the transporter may be modulated, usually by phosphorylation or dephosphorylation reactions; or transport activity can be modified by the rapid insertion or removal of transport proteins from their functional site in the membrane by a process of vesicular exocytosis and/or endocytosis. The latter process involves a change in the number of proteins residing at their functional site, and is increasingly recognized as a mechanism for regulating membrane transport function in a variety of cell systems[2]. Accumulating evidence suggests that transport of bile acids and other organic anions from the liver into bile may also be regulated in part by the targeting of vesicles containing canalicular transporters to the canalicular domain. In this brief review we will summarize the growing evidence that supports this conclusion. To date much of the evidence is circumstantial, and it should be recognized that ultimate proof of these concepts will depend on the development of techniques for quantitation of carrier proteins at the canalicular domain, and correlating functional changes in canalicular transport with quantitative changes in the number of carriers in the membrane. Nevertheless, considerable functional data are accumulating that support such conclusions[3].

To begin with, it is generally accepted that most if not all canalicular proteins are targeted to the apical domain by indirect pathways after first being translocated from the endoplasmic reticulum and Golgi apparatus to the basolateral, sinusoidal domain[4,5]. In this respect the liver cell appears to differ from other polarized epithelia such as the MDCK cell, where apical proteins may be targeted by both direct and indirect pathways[6]. The translocation of proteins from basolateral to apical regions of the hepatocyte is a vesicular process which occurs after endocytic vesicles fuse with, and then bud from, early endosomes. These vesicles move transcytotically attached to microtubules[7]. Intact microtubules have been shown to be essential for canalicular targeting of proteins since microtubule inhibitors block the targeting of proteins to the canalicular domain[8–10]. While previous studies have suggested that microtubule inhibitors have little if any effect on endogenous rates of bile formation in the whole animal (rat), the same treatment blocks excretion of superphysiological infusions of bile acids, as well as physiological levels if the bile acid pool is first depleted[11,12]. Subsequent studies indicate that microtubule dependency for bile acid excretion is more pronounced for hydrophobic as opposed to hydrophilic bile acids[13], implying that physical properties which influence membrane associations may also be important. Similar effects of microtubule inhibitors on biliary excretion have been described for non-bile salt organic anions[14,15].

While these studies can be interpreted to indicate that vesicle targeting to the apical domain may be required to sustain normal canalicular excretory function of organic anions, more recent studies suggest that canalicular membrane transport activity of the Cl^-/HCO_3^- exchanger is also dependent on recruitment of vesicles containing these functional transporters. This process is stimulated by both pH and DBcAMP, and inhibited by phorbol esters[16]. The activity of this exchanger in isolated subconfluent monolayers of rat hepatocytes is enhanced by preincubation in HCO_3^- as opposed to an L-15 medium that is nominally HCO_3^--free. This phenomenon is blocked by colchicine but not by the inactive analogue, lumicolchicine. DBcAMP stimulation of the exchanger is also blocked by colchicine, as well as phorbol esters. This microtubule dependency of Cl^-/HCO_3^- exchanger activation can be reproduced in the isolated perfused rat liver where acute alkalinization stimulates bile flow and bicarbonate excretion, as well as the biliary excretion of the fluid phase marker, horseradish peroxidase[17]. Pretreatment with microtubule inhibitors blocks all three phenomena[17], indicating that activation of this exchanger must require microtubule-dependent fusion of vesicles with the apical domain. Although antibodies to the Cl^-/HCO_3^- exchanger in rat liver have not been available, confocal fluorescent studies performed with antibodies to a canalicular Ca^{2+}, Mg^{2+}-ecto-ATPase suggest that both DBcAMP and preincubation in HCO_3^- media enhance apical translocation of this protein in isolated rat hepatocyte couplets[16]. DBcAMP has also been shown previously to stimulate transcytosis and the biliary excretion of horseradish peroxidase using morphometric measurements in isolated perfused rat liver preparations, a process that again is blunted by microtubule inhibitors[18].

These findings led to more recent studies re-examining whether bile acid transport activity might also be modulated by vesicle targeting. We had previously observed, by video microscopy and optical sectioning, that taurocholate stimulates secretion (luminal expansion) in isolated hepatocyte couplets in proportion to the surface area of the canalicular membrane, rather than the concentration of bile acids in the media[19]. This finding could be explained if there were more bile acid transporters in the couplets with greater canalicular surface areas. Alternatively, the greater canalicular membrane surface area could allow for more osmotic filtration. To assess this question further, studies were conducted which enabled the simultaneous quantitation of canalicular membrane perimeters and functional capacity for bile acid transport by utilizing fluorescent bile acid analogues and quantitative confocal fluorescent imaging. These experiments demonstrated that DBcAMP increased, whereas microtubule inhibitors decreased, the size of the perimeter of the canalicular membrane. These structural changes, which are interpreted to represent stimulation and inhibition of vesicle fusion with the canalicular membrane, correlated closely with quantitative measurements of the functional capacity of the hepatocyte couplets to secrete fluorescent bile acids into the canalicular lumen[20]. These data support the view that changes in the canalicular surface membrane reflect changes in the number of bile acid transporters. While definitive proof of this conclusion must await cloning of the canalicular bile acid transporters, and development of antibodies to these proteins, additional studies have demonstrated that DBcAMP stimulates translocation of the canalicular ecto-ATPase, a putative bile acid transporter[21,22], from cytosol to the apical domain (unpublished observations).

Other studies in the isolated perfused rat liver also support similar conclusions. Swelling of hepatocytes in hypotonic media stimulates exocytosis of vesicles at the canalicular domain in association with an enhancement of physiological rates of bile acid excretion[23] and an increase in the transport maximum for canalicular bile acid transport[24]. Microtubule inhibitors block the effects of volume regulation on vesicle-mediated excretion of the fluid-phase marker, horseradish peroxidase, and also prevent the associated stimulation of biliary bile acid excretion[23,25].

Canalicular transporters for other organic anions may also be regulated by vesicle traffic to the canalicular domain, as recently described in preliminary studies that assess the functional capacity of the canalicular multiple organic anion transporter (cMOAT)[26]. Taken together, all of these observations provide increasing support for the general hypothesis that the bile excretory capacity of the liver is a highly regulated process that depends on the targeting of transcytotic vesicles, containing transport proteins to the canalicular membrane, where they modulate this excretory process by insertion or retrieval from this apical domain.

Acknowledgements

This work was supported by grants DK 25636 and DK 34989, from the National Institutes of Health, USPHS.

References

1. Boyer JL, Graf J, Meier PJ. Hepatic transport systems regulating pHi, cell volume, and bile secretion. Annu Rev Physiol. 1992;54:415–38.
2. Bradbury NA, Bridges RJ. Role of membrane trafficking in plasma membrane solute transport. Am J Physiol. 1994;267:C1–24.
3. Boyer JL. The role of vesicle transport and exocytosis in bile formation and cholestasis: influence of cell volume, pHi, hormones and bile acids. In: Gentilini P *et al.*, editors. Cholestasis. Amsterdam: Elsevier; 1994:69–78.
4. Bartles JR, Feracci HM, Stieger B, Hubbard AL. Biogenesis of the rat hepatocyte plasma membrane *in vivo*: comparison of the pathways taken by apical and basolateral proteins using subcellular fractionation. J Cell Biol. 1987;105:1241–51.
5. Hubbard AL, Stieger B, Bartles JR. Biogenesis of endogenous plasma membrane proteins in epithelial cells. Annu Rev Physiol. 1989;51:755–70.

6. Barroso M, Sztul ES. Basolateral to apical transcytosis in polarized cells is indirect and involves BFA and trimeric G Protein sensitive passage through the apical endosome. J Cell Biol. 1994;124:83–100.
7. Geuze HJ, Slot JW, Strous G.JAM *et al*. Intracellular receptor sorting during endocytosis: comparative immunoelectron microscopy of multiple receptors in rat liver. Cell. 1984;37:195–204.
8. Goldman IS, Jones AL, Hradek CT, Huling S. Hepatocyte handling of immunoglobulin A in the rat: the role of microtubules. Gastroenterology. 1983;85:130–40.
9. Hoppe CA, Connolly TP, Hubbard AL. Transcellular transport of polymeric IgA in the rat hepatocyte: biochemical and morphological characterization of the transport pathway. J Cell Biol. 1985;101:2113–23.
10. Musil LS, Baenziger JU. Proteolytic processing of rat liver membrane secretory component. J Biol Chem. 1988;263:15799–808.
11. Crawford JM, Berken CA, Gollan JL. Role of the hepatocyte microtubular system in the excretion of bile salts and biliary lipid: implications for intracellular vesicular transport. J Lipid Res. 1988;29:144–56.
12. Crawford JM, Gollan JL. Hepatocyte cotransport of taurocholate and bilirubin glucuronides: role of microtubules. Am J Physiol. 1988;255:G121–31.
13. Crawford JM, Strahs DCJ, Crawford AR, Barnes S. Role of bile salt hydrophobicity in hepatic microtubule-dependent bile salt secretion. J Lipid Res. 1994;35:1738–48.
14. Aoyama N, Tokamo H, Ohya T, Chandler K, Holzbach RT. A novel transcellular transport pathway for non-bile salt cholephilic organic anions. Am J Physiol. 1991;261:G305–11.
15. Crawford JM, Gollan JL. Transcellular transport of organic anions in hepatocytes. Hepatology. 1991;14:192–7.
16. Benedetti A, Strazzabosco M, Ng OC, Boyer JL. Regulation of activity and apical targeting of the Cl^-/HCO_3^- exchanger in rat hepatocytes. Proc Natl Acad Sci USA. 1994;91:792–6.
17. Bruck R, Benedetti A, Strazzabosco M, Boyer JL. Intracellular alkalinization stimulates bile flow and vesicular-mediated exocytosis in IPRL. Am J Physiol. 1993;265:G347–53.
18. Hayakawa T, Bruck R, Ng OC, Boyer JL. DBcAMP stimulates vesicle transport and HRP excretion in isolated perfused rat liver. Am J Physiol. 1990;259:G727–35.
19. Gautam A, Ng OC, Strazzabosco M, Boyer JL. Quantitative assessment of canalicular bile formation in isolated hepatocyte couplets using microscopic optical planimetry. J Clin Invest. 1989;83:565–73.
20. Boyer JL, Soroka CL. Vesicle targeting to the apical domain regulates bile secretory function in isolated rat hepatocytes. Gastroenterology. (in press).
21. Sippel CJ, McCollum MJ, Perlmutter DH. Bile acid transport by the rat liver canalicular bile acid transport ecto-ATPase protein is dependent on ATP but not on its own ecto-ATPase activity. J Biol Chem. 1994;269:2820–6.
22. Sippel CJ, Suchy FJ, Ananthanarayanan M, Perlmutter DH. The rat liver ecto-ATPase is also a canalicular bile acid transport protein. J Biol Chem. 1993;268:2083–91.
23. Bruck R, Haddad P, Graf J, Boyer JL. Regulatory volume decrease stimulates bile flow, bile acid excretion, and exocytosis in isolated perfused rat liver. Am J Physiol. 1992;262:G806–12.
24. Haussinger D, Hallbrucker C, Saha N, Lang F, Gerok W. Cell volume and bile acid excretion. Biochem J. 1992;288:681–90.
25. Haussinger D, Saha N, Hallbrucker C, Lang F, Gerok W. Involvement of microtubules in the swelling-induced stimulation of transcellular taurocholate transport in perfused rat liver. Biochem J. 1993;291:355–60.
26. Roelofsen H, Soroka CJ, Boyer JL. Cyclic AMP stimulates sorting of the canalicular multispecific organic ion transporter into the transcytotic bile secretory pathway in hepatocyte couplets. Hepatology. 1994;20:174A.

13
Effects of bile acids on bile duct epithelial cells

M. STRAZZABOSCO, A. ZSEMBERY, A. GRANATO, C. POCI,
A. ROSSANESE and G. CREPALDI

INTRODUCTION

Primary hepatocellular bile is extensively modified while flowing through the biliary system by secretion and/or reabsorption of fluid, electrolytes and other solutes[1,2]. The intrahepatic portion of the bile duct epithelium (BDE) secretes Cl^- and HCO_3^-, both spontaneously and after stimulation with secretin[3,4].

The mechanisms of HCO_3^- secretion by BDE have been extensively studied in cultured cholangiocytes[2,5]. According to the proposed working model, basolateral Na^+/H^+ exchange and $Na : HCO_3$ cotransport mediate HCO_3^- influx into the cell driven by the sodium gradient and the intracellular electric potential[5,6]. The major HCO_3^- efflux mechanism is an apical Cl/HCO_3 exchange (so-called AE-2), the activity of which is stimulated by cAMP and secretin[5,6]. AE-2 stimulation is secondary to the opening of a cAMP-activated Cl^- channel whith electrophysiological properties similar to that of the cystic fibrosis transmembrane conductance regulator (CFTR), that is also expressed at the apical pole of BDE[7–9]. Thus, secretin would stimulate hydrocholeresis by binding to its plasma membrane receptor, followed by an increase in cAMP concentration and by activation of CFTR; Cl^- efflux would then increase the out to in Cl^- gradient, thus favouring HCO_3^- secretion via Cl/HCO_3 exchange.

BDE cells are physiologically exposed to high concentrations of bile acids from the luminal side; however, the effects of bile acids on BDE cells and the role of BDE on bile acid transport and metabolism have received little attention so far. Available information suggests that the bile duct epithelium participates in the 'cholehepatic circulation' of bile acids by passively reabsorbing unconjugated dihydroxy-bile acids that are then glycoconjugated and tauroconjugated and excreted from the basolateral side to the peribiliary circulation. In addition, some bile acids can be toxic for BDE and stimulate BDE proliferation and portal fibrosis.

Alterations in BDE cell transport functions may contribute to the pathogenesis of some cholestatic disorders. In cystic fibrosis, a genetic disease caused by a mutation in the gene encoding for an apical Cl^- channel (CFTR), which is also expressed in the biliary epithelium, hepatobiliary complications occur in about 20% of patients surviving up to 20 years[10]. Interestingly, ursodeoxycholic acid (UDCA.) administration has been reported to improve liver function tests in patients with cystic fibrosis-related liver disease[11], and in patients with primary biliary cirrhosis[12], a chronic cholestatic liver disease primarily affecting the intrahepatic bile duct epithelium.

CHOLEHEPATIC CIRCULATION OF BILE ACIDS

Some unconjugated dihydroxy-bile acids, such as UDCA, stimulate bile flow in excess of that expected from their osmotic activity. 'Hypercholeretic' bile acids also possess the unique property of increasing biliary HCO_3^- concentration and output[13–15].

In isolated rat hepatocyte couplets (IRHC) an experimental model in which events occurring at the bile canalicular level can be selectively studied and dissected from phenomena occurring at the bile duct level[16], administration of UDCA does not increase canalicular expansion rates as compared to TCA, a non-hypercholeretic bile acid[17]. In addition, administration of UDCA to IRHC does not increase canalicular pH, again suggesting that hypercholeresis and biliary HCO_3^- do not originate from the hepatocyte, but must be generated in the bile duct system[18].

Theoretically, UDCA could stimulate HCO_3^- secretion into the bile duct lumen by passive diffusion of protonated UDCA through the biliary epithelium, as predicted by the cholehepatic shunt hypothesis[19–21] or by increasing the activity of specific acid/base transporters in BDE Based on postulated acid/base carrier polarity in bile duct epithelial cells[5], UDCA could increase intracellular HCO_3^- concentration by stimulating Na^+/H^+ exchange, or increase basolateral HCO_3^- influx through $Na : HCO_3$ cotransport activation, or stimulate apical HCO_3^- efflux, by activating Cl/HCO_3 exchange.

We have directly measured the effects of UDCA on intracellular pHi homeostasis in a bile duct epithelium-like cell line[22]. In this model, high doses of UDCA did not stimulate the activity of major carriers involved in acid/base homeostasis (Na^+/H^+ exchange, Na-dependent and -independent Cl/HCO_3 exchange). Rather, similar to what has been previously reported in isolated rat hepatocytes[18,23], UDCA induced a dose-dependent intracellular acidification when administered in the absence of HCO_3^- from the perfusion medium. Acidification was not prevented by furosemide or DIDS, and was deeper in the presence of amiloride. UDCA also caused intracellular acidification of similar degree in fibroblasts, a cell type without transport competence for this bile acid.

These data clearly indicate that UDCA behaves as a permeant weak acid and enters the biliary epithelium, by non-ionic diffusion of its protonated species[24]. Once inside the cell, protonated UDCA will release H^+ ions, as dictated by its pKa, thus decreasing pHi. Administration of a weak organic acid with similar pKa, such as propionate, induced similar changes in pHi, but, because of its lower partion coefficient, 10 times higher concentrations of propionate were needed to achieve a comparable intracellular acidification.

These data are consistent with the cholehepatic shunt hypothesis[19–21]. According to this model, UDCA secreted into the bile in anionic form acquires a proton from carbonic acid at the bile duct level. Biliary HCO_3^- is thus generated by protonation of UDCA anion into the bile duct lumen and by non-ionic diffusion of protonated UDCA. Once reabsorbed, UDCA enters the peribiliary circulation and is carried back to the hepatocytes. Serial recyclings of protonated UDCA would produce hypercholeresis and increased HCO_3^- output.

If not secreted by the biliary epithelium, biliary HCO_3^- must be generated into the biliary lumen by CO_2 hydration. Interestingly, acetazolamide reduces UDCA-stimulated biliary HCO_3^- secretion by 51%[15]. A luminally oriented carbonic anhydrase must therefore be present at the apical pole of cholangiocytes.

BILE ACID METABOLISM AND TRANSPORT BY BDE

Studies with isolated rat common bile ducts demonstrated that the biliary epithelium is in fact able to reabsorb UDCA from the bile and to recirculate it back to the hepatocyte[25]. Having entered the cholangiocyte by non-ionic diffusion, the bile acid will release a proton forming the membrane-impermeant UDCA anion. The cholehepatic circulation therefore requires the presence in cholangiocytes of a bile acid carrier able to extrude UDCA or its conjugates from the basolateral side of the cell.

Although unable to synthesize bile acids from cholesterol, BDE cells can metabolize exogenous bile acids into more polar metabolites[26]. Cultured rat BDE cells conjugate deoxycholic acid, ursodeoxycholic acid and lithocholic acid to glycine and taurine.

Data suggesting the presence in cholangiocytes of a conjugated bile acid carrier have been recently reported, by measuring the uptake of a fluorescent bile acid derivative (NBD-cholyl-*N*-lysine)[27]. Uptake of the bile acid derivative in rat bile duct units (a preparation of cultured small intrahepatic bile ducts) was temperature-dependent, Na-independent, Cl-dependent and DIDS-inhibitable. This basolateral transporter may facilitate conjugated bile acid extrusion from the cholangiocyte into the peribiliary plexus.

EFFECTS OF BILE ACIDS ON INTRACELLULAR SECOND MEDIATORS IN BDE

Bile acids stimulate water and electrolyte secretion from the colonic epithelium. This effect is shared by dihydroxy-bile acids possessing both hydroxy groups in the alpha position (interestingly, they do not include UDCA which has one of its hydroxy groups in the beta position)[28]. Administration of taurodeoxycholate to a colonic epithelial cell line (T84) increases intracellular Ca^{2+} levels and activates a Cl^- conductance[29]. Administration of tauroursodeoxycholic acid (TUDCA) to cultured rat hepatocytes, at physiological concentrations, induce a marked and sustained increase in Ca^{2+} from both intracellular and extracellular sources[30].

The effects of bile acids on intracellular Ca^2 homeostasis have not yet been clearly addressed in BDE cells. A recent preliminary study reported that high doses of UDCA increased intracellular Ca^{2+} levels in biliary cell lines[31], an effect associated with the stimulation of Cl^- efflux from the cell. Although calcium-mobilizing agents increase Cl^- efflux from BDE cells by opening Ca^{2+}-activated Cl^- channels[32], this effect is probably not relevant for hypercholeresis and biliary alkalinization since Cl/HCO_3 exchange activity is not increased by UDCA[22,33]. On the other hand, UDCA-induced Cl^- efflux from BDE might be helpful in cystic fibrosis-related liver disease (in this condition apical Cl^- channels are in fact insensitive to stimulation by cAMP).

In most epithelial cells, changes in intracellular pHi influence a number of cell functions, from volume control to ion secretion and mitosis. However UDCA-induced BDE cell pHi acidification probably has no physiological role since, in the presence of HCO_3/CO_2, acidification is minimal[22,33].

BILE ACIDS AND BDE DAMAGE AND PROLIFERATION

The BDE is a potential target for bile acid toxicity. Disruption of the *mdr2* gene in the mouse, resulting in absence of phospholipids from the bile, is associated with ductular damage and proliferation, probably because the unrestrained detergent effect of high monomeric concentrations of bile acid causes BDE cell damage and inflammation[34]. Chronic administration of lithocholate causes bile duct hyperplasia and portal fibrosis in rats; a single oral dose of lithocholate increases DNA synthesis in the mouse biliary epithelium[35].

Lithocholic acid administration to bile ducts in culture has toxic effects and does not increase the DNA labelling index[36]. Bile duct hyperplasia and fibrosis may thus be secondary to bile acid-induced release of inflammatory mediators from fibroblasts and immune cells in the portal space. It has been shown that BDE cells secretes interleukin 6 (IL-6) after stimulation with interleukin 1β (IL-1β[37]). Interestingly IL-6 is able to stimulate DNA synthesis by BDE cells[37], thus establishing a link between portal inflammation and BDE growth.

Acknowledgements

The authors express their gratitude to Professor L. Okolicsanyi, Dr J. L. Boyer and Dr A. Benedetti for stimulating discussion. A. Z. was a recipient of an International Fellowship from the University of Padova. This work was supported by grant 94.02908.CT04 from the Consiglio Nazionale delle Ricerche and from the 'Centro per lo Studio dell' Invecchiamento'.

References

1. Tavoloni N. The intrahepatic biliary epithelium: an area of growing interest in hepatology. Sem Liver Dis. 1987;7:280–92.
2. Strazzabosco M, Okolicsanyi L, Boyer JL. Acid/base transport systems in isolated bile duct epithelial cells. In: Gentilini P, Dianzani, MU, editors. Experimental and clinical hepatology. Amsterdam: Elsevier; 1991:133–41.
3. Alpini G, Lenzi R, Sarkozi L, Tavoloni N. Biliary physiology in rats with bile ductular cell hyperplasia evidence for a secretory function of proliferated bile ductules. J Clin Invest. 1988;81:569–78.

4. Alpini G, Lenzi R, Zhai W-R, *et al.* Bile secretory function of intrahepatic biliary epithelium in the rat. Am J Physiol. 1989;257:G124–33.
5. Strazzabosco M, Mennone A, Boyer JL. Intracellular pHi regulation in isolated rat bile duct epithelial cells. J Clin Invest. 1991;87:1503–12.
6. Alvaro D, Cho WK. Mennone A, Boyer JL. Effect of secretin on intracellular pH regulation in isolated rat bile duct epithelial cells. J Clin Invest. 1993;92:1314–25.
7. Fitz JG, Basavappa S, McGill J, Melhus O, Cohn JA. Regulation of membrane chloride currents in rat bile duct epithelial cells. J Clin Invest. 1993;91:319–28.
8. McGill J, Basavappa S, Fitz JG. Characterization of high conductance anion channels in rat bile duct epithelial cells. Am J Physiol. 1992;262:G703–10.
9. McGill J, Gettys TW, Basavappa S, Fitz JG. Secretin activates Cl channels in bile duct epithelial cells through a cAMP-dependent mechanism. Am J Physiol. 1994;266:G731–736.
10. Lindblad A, Hultcrantz R, Strandvik B. Bile duct destruction and collagen deposition: a prominent ultrastructural feature of the liver in cystic fibrosis. Hepatology. 1992;16:372–81.
11. Colombo C, Crosignani A, Assaisso M *et al.* Hepatobiliary disease in cystic fibrosis. Hepatology. 1992;16:924–30.
12. Poupon RE, Poupon R, Balkau B and the UDCA–PBC Study group. Ursodiol for the long-term treatment of primaty biliary cirrhosis. N Engl J Med. 1994;330:1342–7.
13. Dumont M, Erlinger S, Uchman S. Hypercholeresis induced by ursodeoxycholic acid and 7-ketolithocholic acid in the rat: possible role of bicarbonate transport. Gastroenterology. 1980;79:82–9.
14. Garcia-Marrin JJ, Corbic M, Dumont M, de Couet G, Erlinger S. Role of H$^+$ transport in ursodeoxycholate-induced biliary HCO_3-excretion in the rat. Am J Physiol. 1985;249:G335–41.
15. Garcia-Marin JJ, Dumont M, Corbic M, de Couet G, Erlinger S. Effect of acid-base balance and acetazolamide on ursodeoxycholete-induced biliary bicarbonate secretion. Am J Physiol. 1985;248:G20–7.
16. Gautam A, Ng OC, Boyer JL. Isolated rat hepatocyte couplets in short-term culture: structural characteristics and plasma membrane reorganization. Hepatology. 1987;7:216–23.
17. Gautam A, Ng OC, Strazzabosco M, Boyer JL. Quantitative assessment of canalicular bile formation in isolated rat hepatocyte couplets using microscopic optical planimetry. J Clin Invest. 1989;83:565–73.
18. Strazzabosco M, Sakisaka S, Hayakawa T, Boyer JL. Effect of UDCA on intracellular and biliary pH in isolated rat hepatocyte couplets and perfused livers. Am J Physiol. 1991;260:G58–69.
19. Yoon YB, Hagey LR, Hofmann AF, Gurantz D, Michelotti EL, Steinbech JH. Effect of side-chain shortening on the physiological properties of bile acids: hepatic transport and effect on biliary secretion of 23-nor-ursodeoxycholate in rodents. Gastroenterology. 1986;90:837–52.
20. Palmer KR, Gurantz D, Hofman AF, Clayton LM, Hagey LR, Cecchetti S. Hypercholeresis induced by nor-chenodeoxycholate in the biliary fistula rat. Am J Physiol. 1987;252:G219–28.
21. Gurantz D, Hofmann AF. Influence of bile acid structure on bile flow and biliary lipid secretion in the hamster. Am J Physiol. 1984;247:G736–48.
22. Strazzabosco M, Poci C, Spirlì C, Sartori L, Knuth A, Crepaldi G. Effect of ursodeoxycholic acid on intracellular pH in a bile duct epithelium-like cell line. Hepatology. 1994;19:145–54.
23. Anwer MS, Hondalus MK, Atkinson JM. Ursodeoxycholate-induced changes in hepatic Na/H exchange and biliary HCO_3 secretion. Am J Physiol. 1989;257:G371–9.
24. Westwergaard H, Dietschy JM. The uptake of lipids into the intestinal mucosa. In: Andreoli TE, Hoffman JF, Fanestil DD, Schultz SG editors. Physiology of membrane disorders. New York: Plenum; 1986:213–24.
25. Farges O, Corbic M, Dumont M, Maurice M, Erlinger S. Permeability of the rat biliary tree to ursodeoxycholic acid. Am J Physiol. 1989;256:G653–60.
26. Hylemon PB, Bohdan PM, Sirica AE, Heuman DM, Vlahcevic ZR. Cholesterol and bile acid metabolism in cultures of primary rat bile ductular epithelial cells. Hepatology. 1990;11:982–8.
27. Benedetti A, Marucci L, Schteingart CD, Ton-Nu HT, Hofmann AF. Uptake of fluorescent bile acids indicates a basolateral transporter for conjugated bile acid anions in polarized bile duct epithelial cells. Gastroenterology. 1994;106:A865 (abstract).
28. Field M. Bile salt-induced diarrhea: the cellular mechanism. J Clin Invest. 1993;92:2091.
29. Devor DC, Sekar CM, Frizzel RA, Duffey ME. Taurodeoxycholate activates potassium and chloride conductances via an IP-3-mediated release of calcium from intracellular stores in a colonic cell line (T84). J Clin Invest. 1993;92:2173–81.

30. Beuers U, Nathanson MH, Boyer JL. Effects of tauroursodexycholic acid on cytosolic Ca^{2+} signals in isolated rat hepatocytes. Gastroenterology. 1993;104:604–12.
31. Shimokura GH, McGill M, Fitz JG. Ursodeoxycholate activates Cl currents in biliary cells through a Ca-dependent mechanism. Gastroenterology. 1994;106:A983, (abstract).
32. McGill J, Basavappa S, Shimohura GH, Middleton JP, Fitz JG. ATP activates ion permeabilities in biliary epithelial cells. Gastroenterology. 1994;107:236–43.
33. Alvaro D, Mennone A, Boyer JL. Effect of ursodeoxycholic acid on intracellular pH regulation in isolated rat bile duct epithelial cells. Am J Physiol. 1993;265:G783–91.
34. Bagheri SA, Bolt MG, Boyer JL, Palmer RH. Stimulation of thymidine incorporation in mouse liver and biliary tract epithelium by lithocholate and deoxycholate. Gastroenterology. 1978;74:188–92.
35. Smit JJM, Schinkel AH, Oude Elferink RPJ et al. Homozygous disruption of the murine mdr2 p-glycoprotein gene leads to a complete absence of phospholipid from bile and to liver disease. Cell. 1993;75:451–62.
36. Gall JAM, Bhathal PS. Isolation and culture of intrahepatic bile ducts and its application in assessing putative inducers of biliary epithelial hyperplasia. Br J Exp Pathol. 1987;68:501–10.
37. Matsumoto K, Fujii H, Michalopoulos G, Fung JJ, Demetris AJ. Human biliary epithelial cells secrete and respond to cytokines and hepatocyte growth factors in vitro: interleukin-6, hepatocyte growth factor and epidermal growth facto promote DNA synthesis in vitro. Hepatology. 1994;20:376–82.

14
Increased biliary secretion of phospholipids in primary sclerosing cholangitis: another mechanism of action of ursodeoxycholic acid?

A. STIEHL, G. RUDOLPH. P. KLÖTERS-PLACHKY, P. SAUER and L. THEILMANN

POSSIBLE MECHANISMS OF ACTION OF URSODEOXYCHOLIC ACID

Treatment of patients with primary sclerosing cholangitis (PCS) with ursodeoxycholic acid (UDCA) leads to improvement of liver enzymes[1–6], serum bilirubin[5], liver histology[5,6] and possibly also improves survival[7]. The mechanism of action is still unclear. Six principal effects seem possible: (1) change in the balance between hydrophilic and hydrophobic bile acids in favour of less toxic hydrophilic bile acids; (2) direct hepatoprotective effect by incorporation in membranes of the liver cell; (3) decrease of hepatocellular concentrations of hepatotoxic bile acids by decreasing their intestinal absorption and/or increasing their biliary secretion; (4) immuno-modulatory effect; (5) choleretic effect with an increased secretion of potentially toxic substances; (6) increased biliary secretion of phospholipids which form mixed micelles preferentially with endogenous bile acids. After their canalicular secretion bile acids and phospholipids form mixed micelles. This trapping of bile acids prevents damage to the biliary canaliculus[8]. In the present study we examined the possibility that UDCA might influence biliary secretion of phospholipids.

KINETICS OF ENDOGENOUS BILE ACIDS

In PSC the pool sizes of cholic acid and chenodeoxycholic acid are small[9]. The increased plasma concentrations of bile acids are due not to increased pool sizes but to increased spillover from the enterohepatic circulation into the peripheral blood and a decrease of bile acids in the enterohepatic circulation. The decreased pool sizes of bile acids were not due to their decreased hepatic synthesis. In patients with PSC and moderately severe cholestasis the pool sizes were reduced, although the hepatic synthesis rates of endogenous bile acids on average were unchanged in comparison to healthy controls[9]. It can be expected, however, that in more severe cholestasis synthesis rates will be reduced. The fractional turnover rates of cholic acid and chenodeoxycholic acid were somewhat increased, but the difference in comparison to healthy controls was not significant[9]. Since most patients with PSC have ulcerative colitis, with the consequence of increased bile acid losses via the intestine, the tendency towards an increased fractional turnover rate is as expected.

EFFECT OF UDCA ON THE KINETICS OF ENDOGENOUS BILE ACIDS

Following UDCA treatment for 3 months the plasma concentrations of bile acids decreased, but the pool sizes of endogenous bile acids remained small[9], indicating a redistribution of bile acids from the peripheral blood into the enterohepatic circulation. Hepatic synthesis rates of cholic acid increased in all patients (Fig. 1) after UDCA, whereas the synthesis of chenodeoxycholic acid was unchanged. The increased hepatic synthesis of bile acids is probably due to their decreased intestinal absorption, with the consequence of a decreased feedback inhibition[10]. Alternatively the increased hepatic synthesis of bile acids might also be the consequence of the decrease of cholestasis.

The fractional turnover of both cholic and chenodeoxycholic acid increased. The most likely explanation for the increased fractional turnover rates of cholic acid

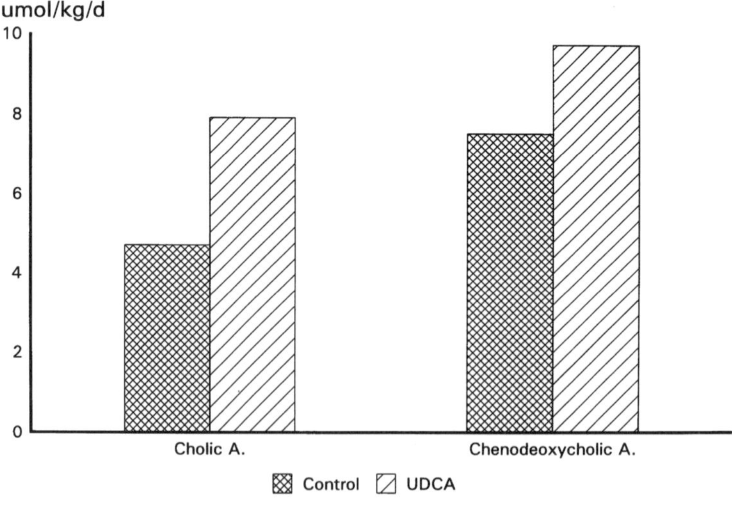

Fig. 1 Effect of ursodeoxycholic acid (UDCA) treatment on the hepatic synthesis rates of cholic acid and chenodeoxycholic acid (from ref. 9). The increase in synthesis of cholic acid was significant ($p < 0.05$), whereas that of chenodeoxycholic acid was not ($p > 0.05$)

and chenodeoxycholic acid after UDCA is the same as for the increased synthesis, namely the fact that UDCA inhibits the absorption of bile acids in the ileum[10].

EFFECT OF UDCA ON BILIARY SECRETION OF BILE ACIDS AND LIPIDS

Following treatment with UDCA, biliary secretion of bile acids increased (Fig. 2), mainly due to an increase in ursodeoxycholic acid secretion[11]. In patients with cholestasis and elevated serum bilirubin secretion of endogenous bile acids was also increased after UDCA[11], indicating improved biliary secretory capacity of the liver after UDCA. The increased biliary secretion of endogenous bile acids was accompanied by a decrease of endogenous bile acids in the peripheral blood. Since the pool sizes of bile acids are unchanged after UDCA[9] these data confirm that there is a redistribution of bile acid pool from the peripheral circulation into the enterohepatic circulation.

The increase in biliary secretion of endogenous bile acids in patients with cholestasis was associated with an increased biliary secretion of cholesterol. The increased biliary secretion of cholesterol is probably responsible for the decrease of plasma cholesterol in cholestatic patients.

After UDCA biliary secretion of phospholipids increased in all patients irrespective of the degree of cholestasis. The correlation coefficient between phospholipid and total bile acid secretion was unchanged. However, the correlation coefficient between phospholipid and endogenous bile acid secretion was increased. Since UDCA dissolves phospholipids and cholesterol very slowly[12], essentially all the phospholipids secreted in the biliary canaliculus will be avail-

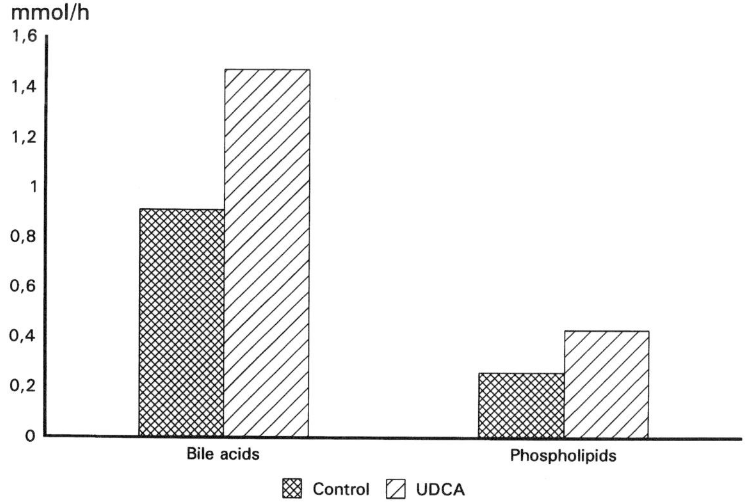

Fig. 2 Effect of ursodeoxycholic acid (UDCA) on biliary secretion of bile acids and phospholipids (from ref. 11). The increase in bile acid secretion ($p < 0.05$) was mainly due to an increased urodeoxycholic acid secretion. The increase in phospholipid secretion was significant ($p < 0.05$)

able for the formation of mixed micelles with endogenous bile acids. The increased biliary secretion of phospholipids may therefore be related tot he beneficial effect of UDCA.

CONCLUSION

Bile-acid-induced liver damage seems to occur primarily in the portal triad[12] where hydrophobic bile acids may solubilize membrane lipids[13]. Among others UDCA may directly stabilize the membrane structure[14]. In addition, phospholipids in the canaliculus may trap toxic, hydrophobic bile acids in mixed micelles, thus detoxifying them. The increase in biliary phospholipid secretion after UDCA treatment[11] may be one of the factors responsible for the protective effect of UDCA at the canalicular site of the hepatocyte.

References

1. Stiehl A, Raedsch R, Kommerell B. The effect of ursodeoxycholic acid in primary sclerosing cholangitis: a comparison to primary biliary cirrhosis. Gastroenterology. 1988;94:A595 (abstract).
2. Hyashi H, Hihuchi T, Ichimiya H, Hishida N, Sakamato N. Asymptomatic primary sclerosing cholangitis: brief report. Gastroenterology. 1990;99:533–5.
3. Chazouilleres O, Poupon R, Capron J-P, *et al.* Ursodeoxycholic acid for primary sclerosing cholangitis. J Hepatol. 1990;11:120–3.
4. O'Brien CB, Senior JR, Arora-Merchandani R, Batta A, Salen G. Ursodeoxycholic acid for the treatment of primary sclerosing cholangitis: a 30 month pilot study. Hepatology. 1991;14:838–47.
5. Beuers U, Spengler U, Kruis W *et al.* Ursodeoxycholic acid for treatment of primary sclerosing cholangitis: a placebo controlled trial. Hepatology. 1992;16:707–14.
6. Stiehl A, Walker S, Stiehl L *et al.* Effect of ursodeoxycholic acid on liver and bile duct disease in primary sclerosing cholangitis. A 3 year pilot study with a placebo controlled study period. J Hepatol. 1994;20:57–64.
7. Stiehl A. Ursodeoxycholic acid therapy in treatment of primary sclerosing cholangitis. Scand J Gastroenterol. 1994;29 (Suppl 204):59–61.
8. Smit JJM, Schinkel AH, Oude Elferink RPJ *et al.* Homozygous disruption of the murine mdr 2-P-glycoprotein gene leads to a complete absence of phospholipid from bile and to liver disease. Cell. 1993;75:451–462.
9. Rudolph G, Endele R, Senn M, Stiehl A. Effect of ursodeoxycholic acid on the kinetics of cholic acid and chenodeoxycholic acid in patients with primary sclerosing cholangitis. Hepatology. 1993;17:1028–32.
10. Stiehl A, Raedsch R, Rudolph G. Acute effects of ursodeoxycholic and chenodeoxycholic acid on the small intestinal absorption of bile acids. Gastroenterology. 1990;98:424–8.
11. Stiehl A, Rudolph G, Sauer P, Theilmann L. Biliary secretion of bile acids and lipids in primary sclerosing cholangitis. Influence of cholestasis and effect of ursodeoxycholic acid treatment. J Hepatol. 1995 (In press).
12. Carey MC, Armstrong MJ, Mazer NA, Igimi H, Savioli G. Measurement of the hydrophilic–hydrophobic balance of bile salts: correlation with physical–chemical interactions between membrane lipids and bile salt micelles. In: Paumgartner G, Stiehl A, Gerok W, editors, Bile acids and cholesterol in health and disease. Lancaster: MTP Press;1983:31–42.
13. Schmucker DL, Ohta M, Kanai S, Sato Y, Kitani K. Hepatic injury induced by bile salts: correlation between biochemical and morphological events. Hepatology. 1990;12:1216–21.
14. Güldütuna S, Zimmer G, Imhof M, Bhatti S, You T, Leuschner U. Molecular aspects of membrane stabilization by ursodeoxycholate. Gastroenterology. 1993;104:1736–44.

15
Bile acid transport systems as pharmaceutical targets: bile acid-derived HMG-CoA reductase inhibitors

W. KRAMER, G. WESS, A. ENHSEN, E. FALK, X.-B. HAN, A. HOFFMANN, G. NECKERMANN and E. PETZINGER

INTRODUCTION

Arteriosclerosis, with its consequences such as myocardial infarction and coronary heart disease, is the major cause of death in western countries. An elevated serum cholesterol level is a major risk factor for arteriosclerosis[1]. The primary therapeutic goal to prevent arteriosclerosis is therefore a decrease of elevated serum LDL-cholesterol levels (Fig. 1). This can be achieved by several approaches such as interruption of the bile acid enterohepatic circulation[2-4], inhibition of intestinal cholesterol absorption[5] or inhibition of hepatic

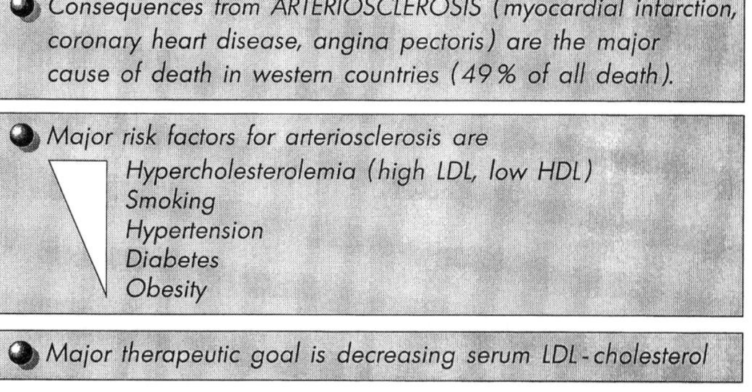

Fig. 1 Characteristics of arteriosclerosis

cholesterol biosynthesis[6]. Cholesterol biosynthesis is a complex biosynthetic event involving more than 20 enzymatic steps[7]. Two enzymes, HMG-CoA synthase and HMG-CoA reductase, are the key enzymes of cholestrol biosynthesis, both being inhibited by the end-product cholesterol in a feedback mechanism[7]. Inhibitors of HMG-CoA reductase – the statins lovastatin, simvastatin and pravastatin – are today the 'gold standard' of lipid therapy. The Scandinavian Simvastatin Survival Study (4S) has recently closed the cholesterol controversy and demonstrated that inhibition of cholesterol biosynthesis dramatically reduces the risk of coronary heart disease (CHD) and improves survival of CHD patients[8].

In 2–5% of patients, however, statins show significant adverse side effects such as elevated liver enzymes[9], severe myositis and rhabdomyolysis[10,11], sleep disturbances[12] and decrease of cardiac ubiquinone levels[13,14]. Extrahepatic actions of the statins are responsible for these side-effects. Since in humans the liver contributes to only 10–20% of body cholesterol biosynthesis[15], but is the major organ for regulation of serum cholesterol levels, an ideal HMG-CoA reductase inhibitor should be active only in the liver and possibly the small intestine[16].

DESIGN OF LIVER-SPECIFIC HMG-CoA-REDUCTASE INHIBITORS

Bile acids undergo an enterohepatic circulation involving the liver and the small intestine under physiological conditions[17–19]. This organotropism of bile acid is established by specific Na^+-dependent transport systems of high transport capacity in hepatocytes[20,21] and ileocytes[22–25].

Protein candidates for the Na^+/bile acid transporters in hepatocytes[26–29] and ileocytes[25,30–32] have been identified by labelling and cloning techniques.

To increase liver-selectivity of HMG-CoA reductase inhibitors we attempted to make use of the physiological transport pathways for bile acids. For this we followed the strategy to combine pharmacophores which are essential for inhibition of HMG-CoA reductase with those of bile acids which are essential for specific uptake by hepatocytes and ileocytes. Two strategies were considered (Fig. 2):

1. Substitution of the bile acid side chain at C-17 against the pharmacophore 3,5-dihydroxyheptanoic acid for inhibition of HMG-CoA reductase to obtain bile acid HMG-CoA reductase inhibitor hybrids which should directly act as enzyme inhibitors.
2. Covalent linkage of conventional HMG-CoA-reductase inhibitors to modified bile acids to obtain prodrugs which should specifically be taken up by hepatocytes with a subsequent intracellular release of the HMG-CoA reductase inhibitor.

The hybrid inhibitors were synthesized with different modifications of the hydroxyl groups at position 7 and 12 of the bile acid moiety, both as lactones and as ring-open acids[33] (Fig. 3). Molecular modelling demonstrates the structural changes of a bile acid molecule by these modifications. The hybrid

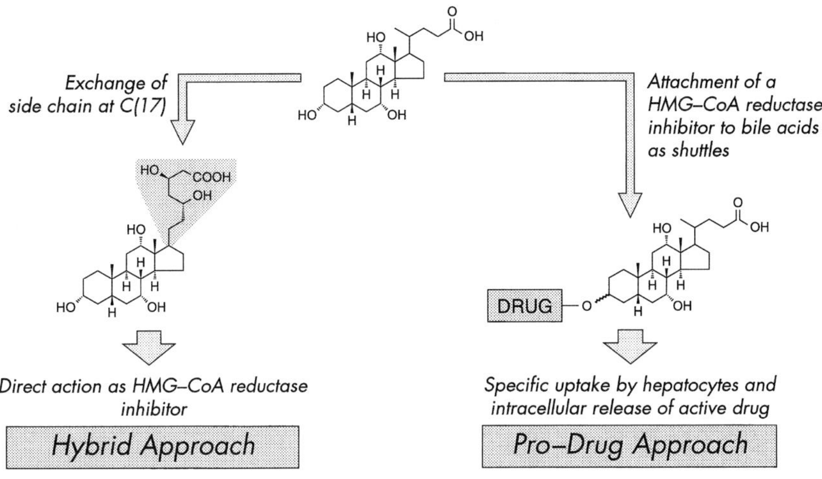

Fig. 2 Strategy of bile acid-derived HMG-CoA reductase inhibitors

molecule is structurally closely related to lovastatin with the additional attachment of *cis*-configurated cyclohexane rings A and B of the steroid nucleus, which are essential structural elements for molecular recognition of a bile acid molecule by bile acid transporters (Fig. 4).

In the prodrugs series the conventional HMG-CoA inhibitors HR 780 and lovastatin were covalently coupled to modified bile acids with linkers of different length, chemical structure and stereochemistry at position 3 of the steroid nucleus[34–37], (Fig. 5). Molecular modelling of these prodrugs shows that the shape of the bile acid moiety in these prodrugs, with about twice the molecular weight of a natural bile acid, is more profoundly conserved than in the hybrids[38].

EFFECT OF BILE ACID-DERIVED HMG-CoA REDUCTASE INHIBITORS ON HMG-CoA REDUCTASE

The hybrid inhibitors stereospecifically inhibited rat liver HMG-CoA reductase. The substituents at the hydroxyl groups 7, and especially 12, of the steroid nucleus had a strong influence on their inhibitory potency. The compounds with a methylbutanoyl function at position 12, which is also present in lovastatin, were most active (Fig. 6, upper panel). The stereospecificity of enzyme inhibition indicates a highly specific interaction of the compounds with HMG-CoA reductase.

The prodrugs were expectantly more than three orders of magnitude less active than the corresponding parent inhibitors, since the free 3,5-dihydroxyheptanoic acid side-chain which is necessary for enzymatic activity as a HMG-CoA reductase inhibitor was masked by attachment of the bile acid (Fig. 6, lower panel). Bile acids such as chenodeoxycholate were inactive as HMG-CoA reductase inhibitors.

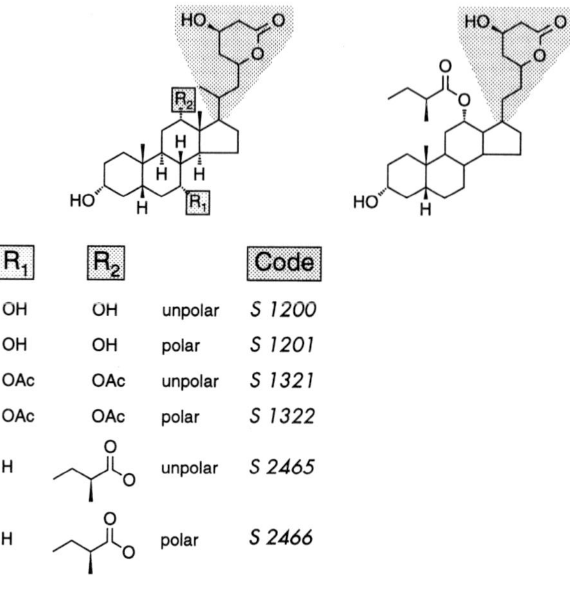

R₁	R₂		Code
OH	OH	unpolar	S 1200
OH	OH	polar	S 1201
OAc	OAc	unpolar	S 1321
OAc	OAc	polar	S 1322
H		unpolar	S 2465
H		polar	S 2466

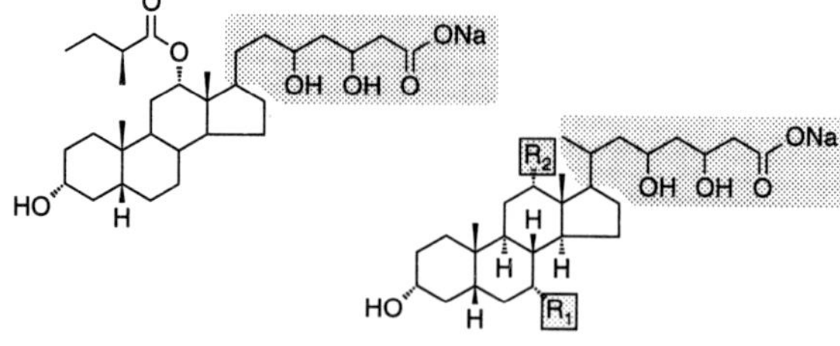

R₁	R₂		Code
OH	OH	unpolar	S 1202
OH	OH	polar	S 1203
OAc	OAc	unpolar	S 1323
OAc	OAc	polar	S 1324
H		unpolar	S 2467
H		polar	S 2468

Fig. 3 Structure of bile acid HMG-CoA reductase inhibitor hybrids

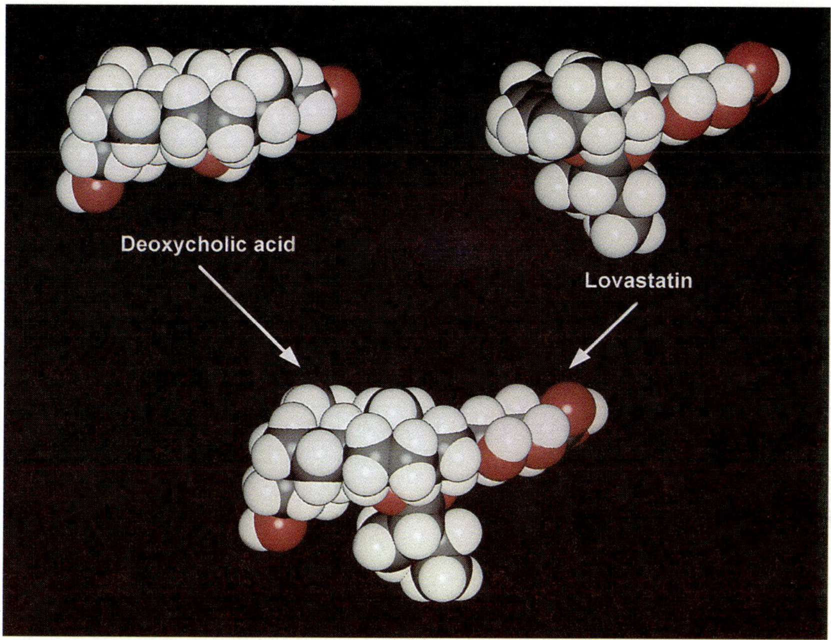

Fig. 4 Space-filling molecular modelling of deoxycholate, lovastatin and the bile acid-derived HMG-CoA reductase inhibitor 21-desmethyl-S 2467

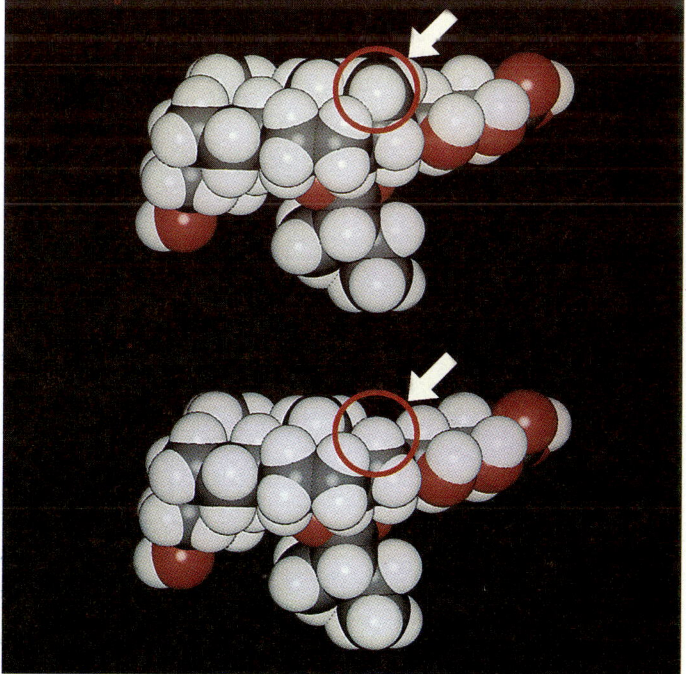

Fig. 10 Space-filling molecular modelling of the bile acid HMG-CoA reductase inhibitor hybrid S 2867 (top) and its 21-desmethyl-derivative (bottom)

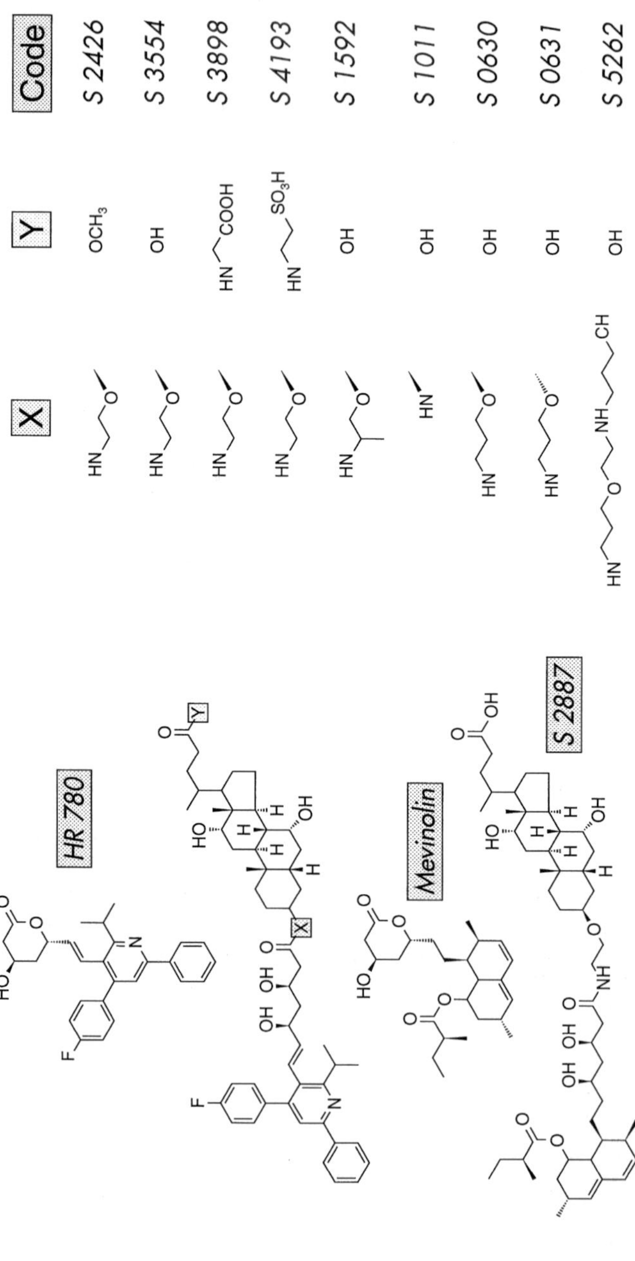

Fig. 5 Structure of bile acid HMG-CoA reductase inhibitor prodrugs

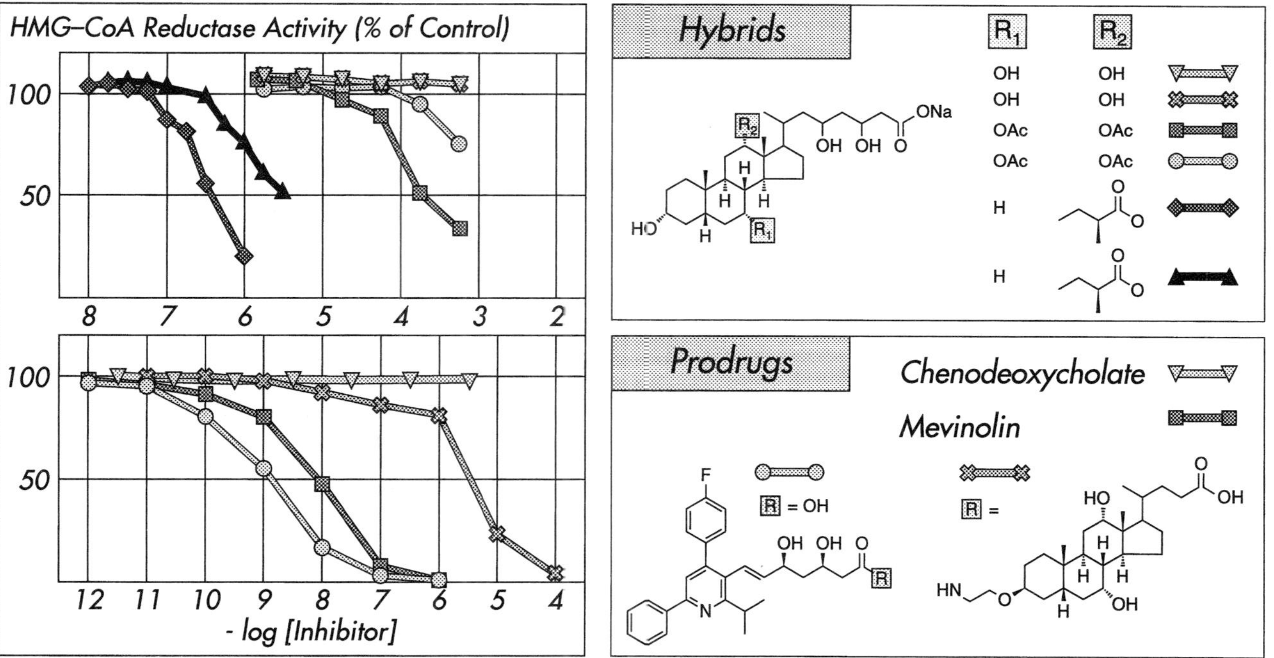

Fig. 6 Effect of bile acid-derived HMG-CoA reductase inhibitors on HMG-CoA reductase from rat liver microsomes. Enzymatic activity of hepatic HMG-CoA reductase in microsomes obtained from rats treated for 10 days with 2% cholestyramine under a reversed light cycle was measured as described[40,42] in the absence or presence of the indicated concentrations of inhibitors

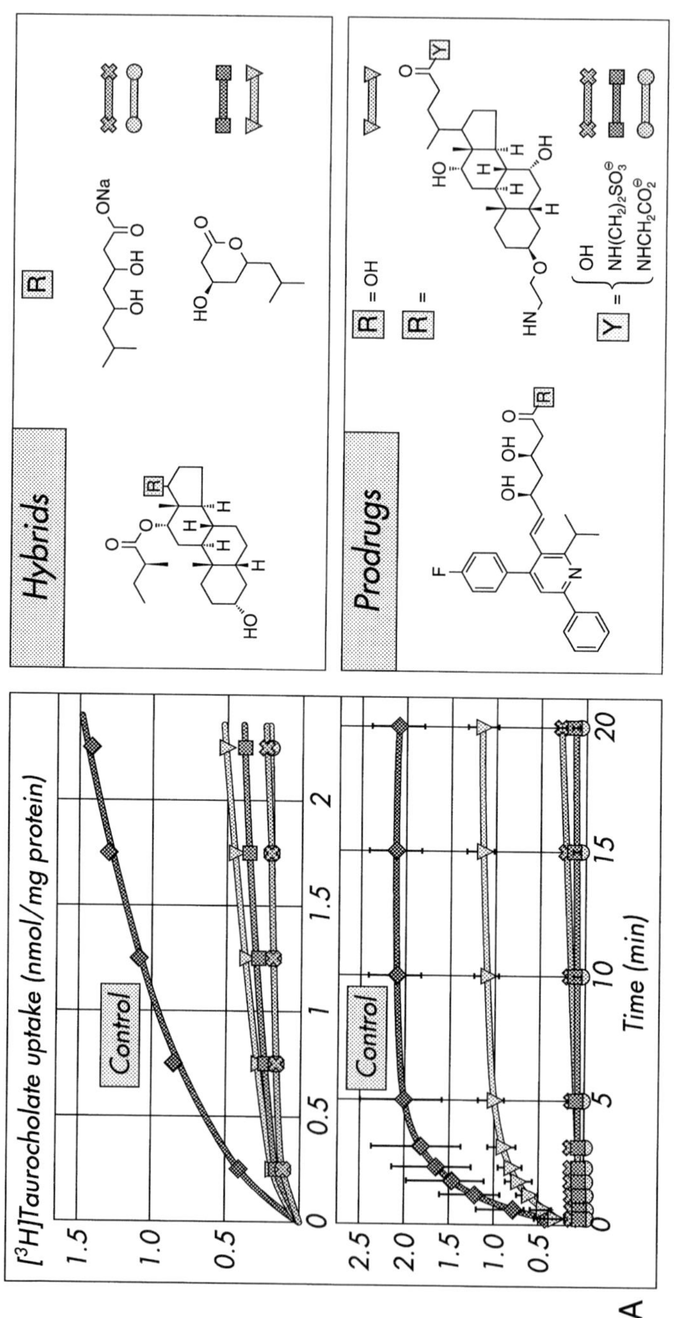

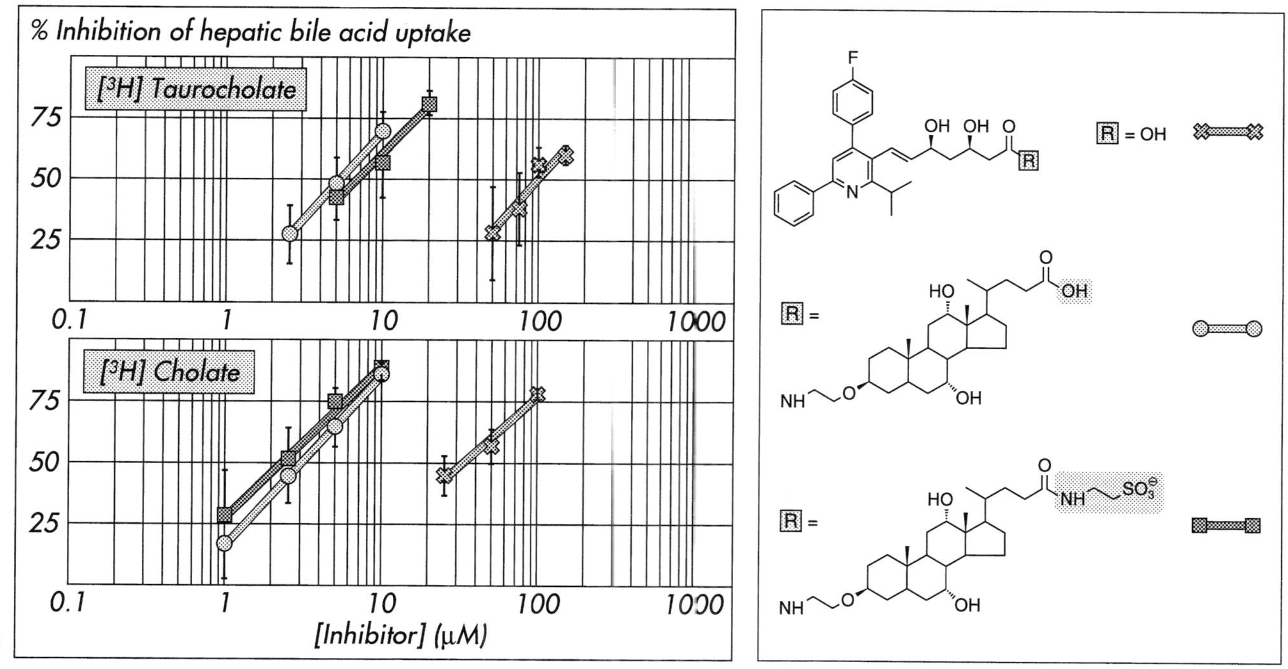

Fig. 7 Inhibition of Na+/[3H]taurocholate uptake into rat hepatocytes by bile acid-derived HMG-CoA reductase inhibitors. Freshly isolated rat hepatocytes[43] (2 × 10^6 cells) suspended in Tyrode buffer were incubated with 100 μmol/l of the indicated compounds for 30 s at 30°C. After addition of 10 μmol/l [3H]taurocholate or 10 μmol/l [14C]cholate, bile acid uptake was measured over the indicated time periods and the amount of radiolabelled bile acids taken up by the cells was measured by the centrifugation method[44]. **A**: Time dependence of [3H]taurocholate uptake. **B**: Concentration-dependence of inhibition of [3H]taurocholate or [14C]cholate uptake by the HMG-CoA reductase inhibitor HR 780 (R = OH) or bile acid derivatives thereof

INTERACTION OF BILE ACID-DERIVED HMG-CoA REDUCTASE INHIBITORS WITH HEPATIC AND ILEAL BILE ACID TRANSPORTERS

To clarify whether the bile acid-derived HMG-CoA reductase inhibitors are recognized by the bile acid transport systems of hepatocytes and ileocytes as substrates, we investigated their effect on taurocholate transport and on photoaffinity labelling of the respective transport proteins. The Na^+-dependent uptake of radiolabelled taurocholate into freshly isolated rat hepatocytes was concentration-dependently inhibited by both series of bile acid-derived HMG-CoA reductase inhibitors (Fig. 7A). If the initial rate of taurocholate uptake was plotted against the concentration of inhibitors, it was obvious that the affinity of a HMG-CoA-reductase inhibitor to the hepatic transporters for taurocholate, as well as for cholate, was increased by more than one order of magnitude after combination with bile acid structural elements (Fig. 7B).

The specificity of bile acid-derived HMG-CoA reductase inhibitors to the hepatocyte bile acid transporters was also shown by photoaffinity labelling. The labelling of the 48 kDa and 54 kDa bile acid-binding proteins in the hepatocyte sinusoidal membrane[26,27,39] was concentration-dependently inhibited by these analogues[40]. In the ileum, Na^+-dependent uptake of radiolabelled taurocholate by brush-border membrane vesicles isolated from rabbit ileum was also concentration-dependently inhibited by both classes of bile acid-derived HMG-CoA-reductase inhibitors, in contrast to conventional HMG-CoA reductase inhibitors which are not recognized by the ileal bile acid transporter showing no inhibitory effect on taurocholate uptake[40]. The prodrugs showed a stronger inhibitory effect, indicating a higher affinity to the ileal bile acid transporter compared to the hybrids. Furthermore, photoaffinity labelling of the protein components of the rabbit ileal bile acid transporter of M_r 93 000 and 14 000[25] was inhibited by the bile acid-derived HMG-CoA reductase inhibitors, whereas conventional HMG-reductase inhibitors such as HR 780 had no significant effect.

A free 3,5-dihydroxyheptanoic acid side-chain of a HMG-CoA reductase inhibitor is essential for optimal activity as an enzyme inhibitor. In the bile acid hybrids hithertho used, the side-chain at carbon 17 of the steroid nucleus still contains a methyl group at position 21. In order to study the influence of the 21-methyl group in HMG-CoA reductase inhibitor bile acid hybrids on the enzymatic activity of HMG-CoA reductase, and on molecular recognition by the ileal bile acid transporter, we synthesized 21-desmethyl compounds. Starting from deoxycholate the desired 21-desmethyl derivatives – which are structurally as close as possible to lovastatin – could be synthesized as pure enantiomers in 18 steps[33] (Fig. 8). The inhibitory potency of the two enantiomers of the 21-desmethyl compounds on HMG-CoA reductase was increased 3-fold (0.2 vs. 0.65 μmol/l) and 7-fold (1.0 vs 7.0 μmol/l) compared to the corresponding 21-methyl derivatives. The affinity to the ileal bile acid transporter, however, decreased by a factor of two (Fig. 9). In contrast to HMG-CoA reductase with a profound stereospecificity of inhibition, the 21-methyl, as well as the 21-desmethyl, derivatives showed (for both enantiomers) an identical affinity to the ileal bile acid transporter. These findings clearly indicate that the methyl group

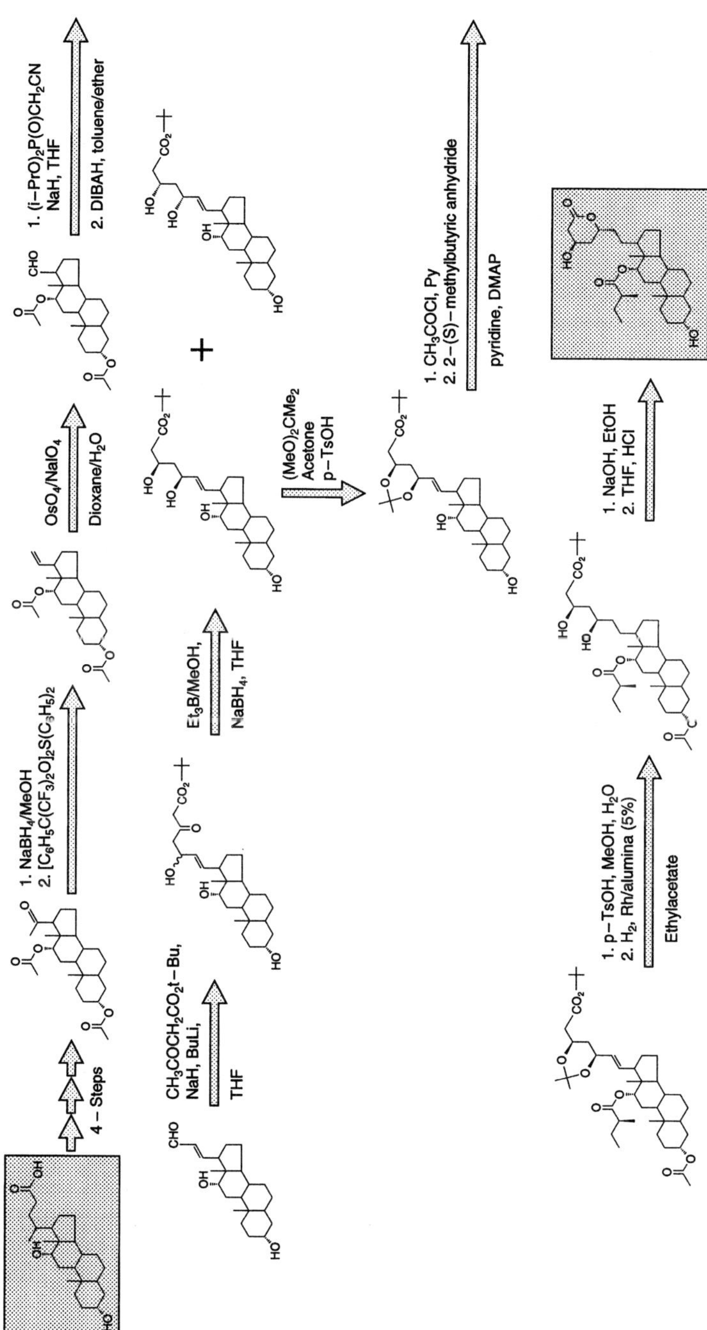

Fig. 8 Synthesis of 21-desmethyl bile acid-derived HMG-CoA reductase inhibitors

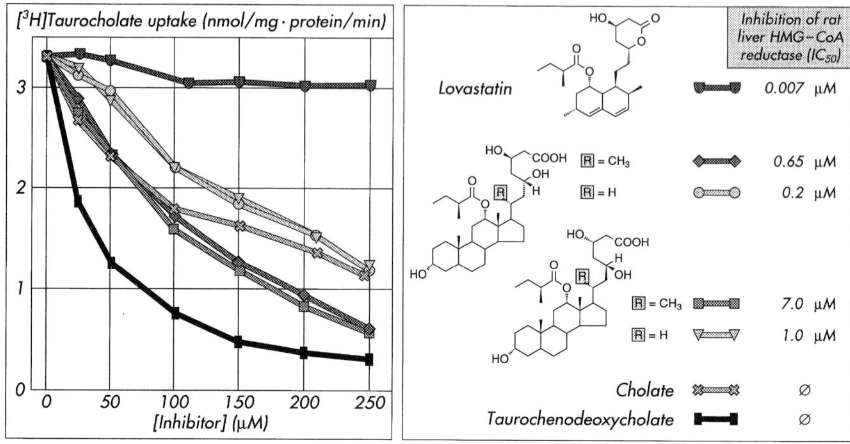

Fig. 9 Effect of 21-methyl and 21-desmethyl bile acid HMG-CoA reductase inhibitor on HMG-CoA reductase and ileal bile acid transport. The inhibitory effect of the indicated compounds on HMG-CoA reductase and IC$_{50}$-values was investigated as described[40,42]. The effect of bile acid-derived HMG-CoA reductase inhibitor hybrids on the ileal bile acid transporter was carried out by incubation of rabbit ileal brush border membrane vesicles (100 μg of protein equilibrated with 10 mmol/l Tris/Hepes buffer ((pH 7.4)/300 mmol/l mannitol) for 60 s with 50 μmol/l [³H]taurocholate solutions in 10 mmol/l Tris/Hepes buffer (pH 7.4)/100 mmol/l NaCl/100 mmol/l mannitol containing the indicated concentrations of inhibitors and subsequent measurement of [³H]taurocholate uptake[45]

at position 21 of the bile acid side-chain significantly contributes to the molecular recognition of a bile acid molecule by the ileal bile acid transporter (Fig. 10).

To demonstrate efficacy of bile acid-derived HMG-CoA reductase inhibitors in cells and living animals, cholestrol biosynthesis in Hep-G2 cells was measured as incorporation of [^{14}C]acetate into cholesterol. Cholesterol biosynthesis was inhibited by the hybrid as well as the prodrug inhibitors. The prodrug S 3554 showed an IC$_{50}$-value of 68 nmol/l compared to about 8 μmol/l on the isolated enzyme or with rat liver microsomes, which indicates a release of the active drug from the prodrug within the Hep-G2 cell. The hybrids were much less potent, showing an IC$_{50}$ value of 2 μmol/l for the best compound – the 21-desmethyl derivative of S 2867 – compared to 30 nmol/l for lovastatin[40].

In order to demonstrate a liver-specific delivery of the prodrug, *in situ* liver perfusion experiments were performed. After bolus injection of HMG-CoA-reductase inhibitors or their corresponding bile acid prodrug, the bile acid conjugate showed a secretion profile into bile similar to a natural bile acid in contrast to the parent HMG-CoA reductase inhibitor HR 780[38,40]. After 1 or 2 hours approximately twice the amount of applied drug was secreted into bile with the bile acid conjugate compared to the parent drug. The secretion profile and the intracellular release of the HMG-CoA reductase inhibitor from the prodrug within the hepatocyte was greatly influenced by the structure of the linker between the drug and the bile acid moiety. With 3-carbon linkers, especially with α-orientation at position 3 of the steroid nucleus, a delayed and long-acting release of the active drug could be achieved (Fig. 11). After intravenous application either of HR 780 or its bile acid conjugate S 3554 the organ distribution of the drugs was measured. The bile

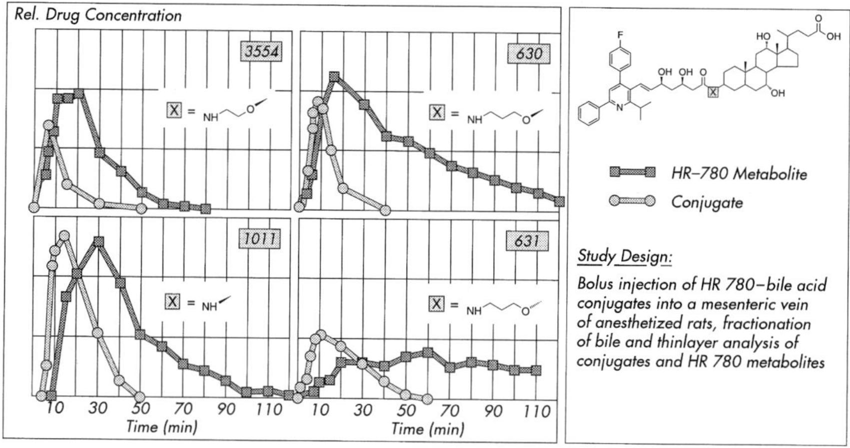

Fig. 11 Influence of the linker in HMG-CoA reductase inhibitor bile acid prodrugs on intracellular release and biliary secretion profile. The HR-780 bile acid conjugates S 3554, S 0630, S 0631 or S 1011, dissolved as 1 mmol/l solutions in 10 mmol/l Tris/Hepes buffer (pH 7.4)/300 mmol/l mannitol/5% ethanol were injected as bolus into a peripheral mesenteric vein of anaesthetized rats. After cannulation of the common bile duct the bile was fractionated and the content of HR 780-bile acid conjugates or metabolites was analysed by thin-layer chromatography[46]

acid conjugate preferably concentrated in the liver and the biliary system with significantly lower concentrations in extrahepatic tissues. After oral application of the bile acid-derived HMG CoA reductase inhibitors to rats, cholesterol biosynthesis in the liver and the small intestine was measured. The bile acid prodrug S 3554 inhibited cholesterol biosynthesis only in the liver, in contrast to lovastatin. Furthermore, the pharmacokinetic profile of lovastatin and the bile acid conjugate S 3554 differed significantly, with a slower onset of inhibition by the bile acid prodrug[40]. This delayed pharmacological action is presumably caused by the intestinal passage time of the prodrug in the small intestine to the terminal ileum, where the intact compound is absorbed via the ileal bile acid transporter. After transport with portal blood to the liver the conjugate is selectively taken up by the hepatocytes, with subsequent intracellular release of the HMG-CoA reductase inhibitor. The concentrations of S 3554 in extrahepatic tissues such as adrenal gland, heart or testicles were up to a factor of 10 lower than with HR 780[40], which itself is a liver-selective HMG-CoA reductase inhibitor[41].

CONCLUSIONS

These investigations clearly demonstrate an improvement of liver selectivity of HMG-CoA reductase inhibitors by combination with structural elements of bile acids.

1. Substitution of the bile acid side-chain at C-17 of the steroid nucleus by 3,5-dihydroxyheptanoic acid side-chain converts bile acids to stereospecific inhibitors of HMG-CoA reductase.

2. Bile acid-derived HMG-CoA reductase inhibitors – both prodrugs and hybrids – are specifically recognized by the hepatocyte and ileocyte bile acid transporters.
3. Bile acid-derived HMG-CoA reductase inhibitors inhibit cholesterol biosynthesis in Hep-G2 cells and the prodrugs also showed oral activity.

Acknowledgements

For their assistance in synthesis and biological experiments the authors are greatly indepted to K. Benstein, K. Bock, J. Dumke, W. Gerlach, F. Girbig, U. Gutjahr, R. Hofmann, B. Karbe-Thönges, R. Kaulfuß v.d. Heyden, H. Kleine, S. Kowalewski, C. Kremer, M. Meyer, M. Schmalz, H.-J. Thönges, R. Watkowiak and B. Worzischek. We thank Mrs Susanne Winkler for excellent secretarial assistance.

References

1. Gotto AM Jr, LaRosa JC, Hunnighake D *et al*. The cholesterol facts. A summary of the evidence relating dietary fats, serum cholesterol, and coronary heart disease. Circulation. 1990;81:1721–33.
2. Benson GM, Hickey DMB. Bile acid sequestrants: past and future. Current Drugs. Anti-atherosclerotic Agents. 1991:B43–59.
3. Wess G, Kramer W, Enhsen A *et al*. Specific inhibitors of ileal bile acid transport. J Med Chem. 1994;37:873–5.
4. Kramer W, Wess G, Baringhaus K-H *et al*. Design and properties of ileal bile acid transport inhibitors. In: Hofmann A, Paumgartner G, Stiehl A, editors. Bile acids in gastroenterology: basic and clinical advances. Dordrecht: Kluwer; 1995:205–220.
5. Harwood HJ Jr, Chandler CE, Pellarin LD *et al*. Pharmacologic consequences of cholesterol absorption inhibition: alteration in cholesterol metabolism and reduction in plasma cholesterol concentration induced by the synthetic saponin β-tigogenin cellobioside (CP-88818; tiqueside). J Lipid Res. 1993;34:377–95.
6. Grundy SM. HMG-CoA reductase inhibitors for treatment of hypercholesterolemia. N Engl J Med. 1988;319:24–32.
7. Goldstein JL, Brown MS. Regulation of the mevalonate pathway. Nature. 1990;343:425–30.
8. Scandinavian Simvastatin Survival Study Group. Randomized trial of cholesterol lowering in 4444 patients with coronary heart disease: the Scandinavian Simvastatin Survival Study (4S). Lancet. 1994;344:1383–9.
9. Henwood JM, Heel RC. Lovastatin. A preliminary review of its pharmacodynamic properties and therapeutic use in hyperlipidemia. Drugs. 1988;36:429–54.
10. Israeli A, Raveh D, Arnon R, Eisenberg S, Stein Y. Lovastatin and elevated creatine kinase: results of rechallenge. Lancet. 1989;1:725.
11. Walravens RA, Greene C, Frerman FE. Lovastatin, isoprenes and myopathy. Lancet. 1989;2:1097–1098.
12. Schaefer E. HMG-CoA reductase inhibitor for hypercholestemia. N Engl J Med. 1988;319:1222.
13. Willis RA, Folkers K, Tucker J-H, Ye C-Q, Xia L-J, Tamagawa M. Lovastatin decreases coenzyme Q levels in rats. Proc Natl Acad Sci USA. 1990;87:8928–30.
14. Folkers K, Langsjoen P, Willis R *et al*. Lovastatin decreases coenzyme Q levels in humans. Proc Natl Acad Sci USA. 1990;87:8531–4.
15. Turley S, Dietschy JM. The metabolism and excretion of cholesterol by the liver. In: Arias IM, Jakoby WB, Popper H, Schachter D, Shavritz DA, editors. Biology and pathobiology, 2nd edn. New York: Raven Press; 1988:pp 617–41.
16. Mosley ST, Kalinowski SS, Schafer BL, Tanaka RD. Tissue-selective acute effects of inhibitors of 3-hydroxy-3-methylglutaryl coenzyme A reductase on cholesterol biosynthesis in lens. J Lipid Res. 1989;30:1411–20.

17. Carey MC, Cahalane MJ. Enterohepatic circulation. In: Arias IM, Jakoby WB, Popper H, Schachter D, Shatritz DA, editors. The liver: biology and pathobiology, 2nd edn. New York: Raven Press; 1988:576–616.

18. Vlachevic ZR, Heuman DM, Hylemon PB. Physiology and pathophysiology of enterohepatic circulation of bile acids. In: Zakim D, Boyer TD editors. Hepatology. Philadelphia: WB Saunders; 1990:341–77.

19. Hofmann AF. Intestinal absorption of bile acids and biliary constituents. The intestinal component of the enterohepatic circulation and the integrated system. In: Johnson LR, editor. Physiology of the gastrointestinal tract, 3rd edn. New York: Raven Press; 1994:1845–65.

20. Anwer MS, Kroker R, Hegner D. Cholic acid uptake into isolated rat hepatocytes. Hoppe-Seyler's Z Physiol Chem. 1976;375:1477–86.

21. Schwarz LR, Burr R, Schwenk M, Pfaff E, Greim H. Uptake of taurocholic acid into isolated rat-liver cells. Eur J Biochem. 1975;55:617–23.

22. Wilson FA. Intestinal transport of bile acids. Am J Physiol. 1991;241:683–92.

23. Lack L. Properties and biological significance of the ileal bile salt transport system. Environ Health Perspect. 1979;33:79–90.

24. Burckhardt G, Kramer W, Kurz G, Wilson FA. Inhibition of bile salt transport in brush-border membrane vesicles from rat small intestine by photoaffinity labeling. J Biol Chem. 1983;258:3618–22.

25. Kramer W, Girbig F, Gutjahr U *et al.* Intestinal bile acid absorption: Na$^+$-dependent bile acid transport activity in rabbit small intestine correlates with the coexpression of an integral 93 kDa and a peripheral 14 kDa bile acid-binding membrane protein along the duodenum-ileum axis. J Biol Chem. 1993;268:18035–46.

26. Kramer W, Bickel U, Buscher HP, Gerok W, Kurz G. Bile acid binding polypeptides in plasma membranes of hepatocytes revealed by photoaffinity labeling. Eur J Biochem. 1982;129:13–24.

27. von Dippe P, Levy D. Characterization of the bile acid transport system in normal and transformed hepatocytes. J Biol Chem. 1983;258:8896–901.

28. Ziegler K, Frimmer M, Fasold H. Further characterization of membrane proteins involved in the transport of organic anions in hepatocytes. Comparison of two different affinity labels: 4,4′-diisothiocyano-1,2-diphenylethane-2.2′-disulfonic acid and brominated taurodehydrocholic acid. Biochim Biophys Acta. 1984;769:117–29.

29. Hagenbuch B, Stieger B, Foguet M, Lübbert H, Meier PJ. Functional expression cloning and characterization of the hepatocyte Na$^+$/bile acid cotransport system. Proc Natl Acad Sci USA. 1991;88:10629–33.

30. Kramer W, Burckhardt G, Wilson FA, Kurz G. Bile salt-binding polypeptides in brush-border membrane vesicles from rat small intestine revealed by photoaffinity labeling. J Biol Chem. 1983;258:3623–7.

31. Kramer W, Nicol S-B, Girbig F, Gutjahr U, Kowalewski S, Fasold H. Characterization and chemical modification of the Na$^+$-dependent bile acid transport system in brush-border membrane vesicles from rabbit ileum. Biochim Biophys Acta. 1992;1111:93–102.

32. Wong MH, Oelkers P, Craddock AL, Dawson PA. Expression cloning and characterization of the hamster ileal sodium-dependent bile acid transporter. J Biol Chem. 1994;269:1340–7.

33. Wess G, Kramer W, Han X-B *et al.* Synthesis and biological activity of bile acid-derived HMG-CoA reductase inhibitors. The role of 21-methyl in recognition of HMG-CoA reductase and the ileal bile acid transport system. J Med Chem. 1994;37:3240–6.

34. Wess G, Kramer W, Bartmann W *et al.* Modified bile acids: preparation of the 7α, 12α-dihydroxy-3β- and 7α, 12α-dihydroxy-3α-(2-hydroxyethoxy)-5β-cholanic acid and their biological activity. Tetrahedron Lett. 1992;33:195–8.

35. Wess G, Kramer W, Schubert G *et al.* Synthesis of bile acid-drug conjugates: potential drug-shuttles for liver specific targeting. Tetrahedron Lett. 1993;34:819–22.

36. Wess G, Kramer W, Enhsen A *et al.* Preparation of 3α- and 3β-(ω-aminoalkoxy)-7α,12α-dihydroxy-5β-cholanoic acid esters: versatile shuttles for drug targeting. Tetrahedron Lett. 1993;34:817–18.

37. Kramer W, Wess G. European Patent Application EP 0417725 A2, 1989.

38. Kramer W, Wess G, Schubert G *et al.* Bile acids as carriers for drugs: In: Paumgartner G, Stiehe A, Gerok W, editors. Bile acids and the hepatobiliary system. Lancaster: Kluwer; 1993:161–76.

39. Wieland T, Nassal M, Kramer W, Fricker G, Bickel U, Kurz G. Identity of hepatic membrane transport systems for bile salts, phalloidin and antamanide by photoaffinity labeling. Proc Natl Acad Sci USA. 1984;81:5232–6.
40. Kramer W, Wess G, Enhsen A *et al*. Bile acid derived HMG-CoA reductase inhibitors. Biochim Biophys Acta. 1994;1227:137–54.
41. Krause R, Neubauer H, Leven M, Kesseler K. Inhibition of cholesterol synthesis in target tissues and extrahepatic organs after administration of HMG-CoA reductase inhibitors in normolipidemic rats: organ selectivity and time course of the inhibition. J Drug Dev. 1990;3(Suppl. 1):255–7.
42. Ong KK, Khor HT, Than DTS. Assay of 3-hydroxy-3-methylglutaryl CoA reductase activity using anionic-exchange column chromatography. Anal Biochem. 1991;196:211–14.
43. Petzinger E, Seeger R. Scanning electron microscopic studies on the cytolytic effect of phallolysin on isolated rat hepatocytes and AS-30 D hepatoma cells. Naunyn Schmiedeberg's Arch Pharmacol. 1976;295:211–13.
44. Petzinger E, Müller N, Föllmann W, Deutscher J, Kinne RKH. Uptake of bumetanide into isolated rat hepatocytes and primary liver cell cultures. Am J Physiol. 1989;256:G78–86.
45. Kramer W, Wess G, Neckermann G *et al*. Intestinal absorption of peptides by coupling to bile acids. J Biol Chem. 1994;269:10621–7.
46. Kramer W, Wess G, Schubert G *et al*. Liver-specific drug targeting by coupling to bile acids. J Biol Chem. 1992;267:18598–604.

Section V
Ursodeoxycholic acid treatment in cholestatic liver diseases

16
Long-term experience with ursodeoxycholic acid for patients with primary biliary cirrhosis and primary sclerosing cholangitis

K. D. LINDOR

INTRODUCTION

Ursodeoxycholic acid (UDCA) has been shown to be a safe and effective treatment for patients with primary biliary cirrhosis (PBC)[1-3]. Much less information is available about the role of UDCA for patients with primary sclerosing cholangitis (PSC) because of the very small number of patients reported in trials, usually of short duration[4-6]. UDCA, however, remains promising in PSC and is still under investigation in this setting. Information about the long-term effectiveness of UDCA on PBC is limited; although three of the largest randomized trials have had data analysed up to 4 years.

In the French multicentre study a total of 145 patients received a dose of 13–15 mg/kg per day of UDCA or placebo for 2 years[1]. In mid-1994, after all patients had received UDCA for at least 2 years and some up to 4 years, the probability of liver transplantation (or referral) was significantly less in the group that was originally randomized to receive UDCA; similarly, the probability of liver transplantation or death was also significantly lessened in the group receiving UDCA for the full period[7].

In the Canadian multinational trial reported by Heathcote *et al.* 222 patients were randomized to receive approximately 14 mg/kg per day of UDCA or placebo for a 2-year period[2]. One hundred patients in the Toronto area were offered UDCA for an additional 6–24 months afterwards. Ninety patients accepted, 49 of whom had been originally randomized to the UDCA group. The main results of the original study showed that UDCA improved bilirubin, the main endpoint of the study, and there were non-significant trends towards improved survival or avoiding transplantation in the group receiving UDCA. The 4-year follow-up in the 49 patients initially treated with UDCA showed sustained improvement over baseline in liver biochemistries from 2 to 4 years with minimal deterioration of these tests from 2 to 4 years[8].

In our own study of 180 patients receiving 13–15 mg/kg per day, patients were randomized to receive UDCA or placebo over a total period of up to 4 years with a minimum of 2-year follow-up available in 132 patients[3]. In this study, the time until treatment failure (defined as death, transplantation, progression to cirrhosis, development of complications of portal hypertension, voluntary withdrawal, or doubling of bilirubin) was significantly improved in patients receiving UDCA. There was a non-significant trend towards improvement in time until death or transplantation in the group receiving UDCA over this period of study.

The data from the French, Canadian, and Mayo studies described above have been combined in a recently submitted abstract. This analysis compared the survival free of transplantation in groups originally assigned to UDCA versus placebo in the three studies over a 4-year period, and confirmed the results reported by Poupon *et al.*[7] We have also submitted an abstract evaluating our long-term follow up of UDCA treated PBC patients over a 6-year period. We compared the survival of those patients receiving UDCA for up to 6 years with the expected survival based on that predicted by the Mayo Risk Score[9]. The expected survival was corrected for improved baseline care (including the use of liver transplantation) since the model was developed, and showed significant benefit in favour of UDCA.

Lastly, Huet *et al.* have presented data on the long-term effects of UDCA on hepatic function and portal pressure in patients with PBC at 6 years[10]. Patients in this study had a significantly greater increase in portal pressure when treated with placebo. With UDCA the portal hepatic gradient showed a slight rise at 2 years, but returned to baseline at 4 years and was stable at 6 years. These workers concluded that long-term use of UDCA could reverse progression of portal hypertension.

UNANSWERED QUESTIONS

There are a number of questions to be answered about the use of UDCA for patients with PBC. Two of these include criteria for appropriate patient selection and optimal dose.

Patient selection

Jorgensen *et al.* have reported that 19% of UDCA-treated PBC patients have complete and sustained biochemical normalization when receiving a dose of 13–15 mg/kg per day of UDCA[11]. Characteristics of these complete responders include a lower initial alkaline phosphatase (943 versus 1417 u/l), a lower bilirubin (0.7 versus 2.3 mg/dl), and a greater percentage of UDCA in bile at 2 years (56% versus 38%) when compared to those patients receiving UDCA without such a complete response.

At the other end of the scale, Poupon's 4-year follow-up of patients receiving UDCA for PBC, predictors of death in patients receiving UDCA included high bilirubin, low albumin, and splenomegaly[7].

To my knowledge the Mayo study was the only one to report a subgroup analysis of the effects of UDCA in PBC patients with cirrhosis or hyperbilirubinaemia. In patients with cirrhosis or serum bilirubin levels greater than 1.8 mg/dl, the use of UDCA led to significantly improved time to treatment failure compared to placebo, suggesting that even those patients with more advanced disease can derive significant benefit from UDCA[3].

Dosage

There is little information presently available regarding the most appropriate dose of UDCA. In the US multinational study, reported so far only in abstract form, 153 patients received a lower dose of 10–12 mg/kg per day of UDCA[12]. There was no difference in the frequency or time to treatment failure with UDCA versus placebo. Moreover, liver tests were improved only in those with a bilirubin of less than 2 mg/dl.

In a study by Podda in a small number of patients with PBC, liver biochemistries were improved with doses as low as 250 mg per day of UDCA, but there was significantly more improvement with doses of 500 or 750 mg per day[13].

We are currently conducting a trial comparing three different doses of UDCA for PBC in which we will measure the effects on liver biochemistries and biliary enrichment. Over 100 patients are entered and have been randomized to receive doses of 5–7 versus 13–15 versus 23–25 mg/kg per day of UDCA.

URSO FOR PSC

There is minimal long-term data regarding the use of UDCA for PSC. Chazouilleres *et al.* reported 15 patients who received UDCA at a dose of 750–1250 mg per day for 6 months[4]. There was biochemical improvement in these patients with alkaline phosphatase improving from 401 to 222 U/l on average. Three patients voluntarily withdrew from UDCA and had prompt worsening of liver biochemistries with discontinuation.

O'Brien *et al.* reported 12 PSC patients receiving 10 mg/kg per day of UDCA studied over a 30-month period, in which the first 3 months were observation followed by UDCA treatment for 6 months[5]. There was another 3 months of observation off UDCA and then a long-term treatment phase extending out to at least 18 months with UDCA. During the time the UDCA was used, there were improved liver biochemistries which were sustained in some patients for up to 2 years in follow-up.

The only placebo-controlled randomized trial was conducted in 14 patients reported by Beuers *et al.* These patients received 13–15 mg/kg per day of UDCA or placebo, and were followed for 12 months. They had improvement in liver tests and improved histology using a multiparametric score.

Stiehl reported 20 patients who had received 750 mg per day of UDCA for at least 1 year[14]. They were randomized either to continue UDCA or be withdrawn, but this trial was terminated after 3 months because of worsening liver biochemistries in the group withdrawn. Importantly, they did describe biochemical improvement for up to 2 years in these patients studied.

Our own data recently reported, regarding the role of UDCA versus UDCA plus methotrexate, included nine patients receiving UDCA alone who had sustained improvement in liver biochemistries for up to 2 years. The addition of methotrexate appeared to add little benefit, but was associated with toxicity[15].

We are currently nearing conclusion of a trial of UDCA versus placebo for PSC patients. Approximately 100 patients have been entered. The study began in mid-1989, and we plan to conclude in mid-1995, which will provide us data up to 6 years. It is hoped that the results of this study will provide more conclusive information regarding the overall effects of UDCA for patients with PSC, as well as providing substantial information about its long-term use.

SUMMARY

The long-term use of UDCA in PBC is associated with a sustained improvement in liver tests, decreases the need for liver transplantation, and improves survival. UDCA is often considered the treatment of choice for these patients; although it has not yet been approved for this use by the FDA in the United States.

The long-term use of UDCA in PSC remains to be assessed. Up to 2 years of treatment may lead to biochemical improvement, and the overall long-term effects of UDCA in PSC will probably be elucidated in the near future.

References

1. Poupon RE, Balkau B, Eschwege E, Poupon R and the UDCA-PBC Study Group. A multicenter, controlled trial of ursodiol for the treatment of primary biliary cirrhosis. N Engl J Med. 1991;324:1584–54.
2. Heathcote EJ, Cauch-Dudek K, Walker V *et al*. The Canadian multicenter double-blind randomized controlled trial of ursodeoxycholic acid in primary biliary cirrhosis. Hepatology. 1994;19:1149–56.
3. Lindor KD, Dickson ER, Baldus WP *et al*. Ursodeoxycholic acid in the treatment of primary biliary cirrhosis. Gastroenterology. 1994;106:1284–90.
4. Chazouilleres O, Poupon R, Capron JP *et al*. Ursodeoxycholic acid for primary sclerosing cholangitis. J Hepatol. 1990;11:120–3.
5. O'Brien CB, Senior JR, Arora-Mirchandani R, Batta AK, Salen R. Ursodeoxycholic acid for the treatment of primary sclerosing cholangitis: a 30-month pilot study. Hepatology. 1991;14:838–47.
6. Beuers U, Spengler U, Kruis W *et al*. Ursodeoxycholic acid for the treatment of primary sclerosing cholangitis: a placebo-controlled trial. Hepatology 1992;16:707–14.
7. Poupon RE, Poupon R, Balkau B and the UDCA-PBC Study Group. Ursodiol for the long-term treatment of primary biliary cirrhosis. N Eng J Med. 1994;330:1342–7.
8. Heathcote EJL, Cauch K, Walver V *et al*. A four-year follow-up study of ursodeoxycholic acid therapy for primary biliary cirrhosis. Gastroenterology. 1993;104:A914.
9. Dickson ER, Grambsch PM, Fleming TR, Fisher LD, Langworthy A. Prognosis of primary biliary cirrhosis: model for decision making. Hepatology. 1989;10:1–7.
10. Huet PM, Huet J, Hotte S. Long term effect of ursodeoxycholic acid (UDCA) on hepatic function and portal hypertension in primary biliary cirrhosis (PBC). Hepatology. 1994;20:202A.
11. Jorgensen RA, Dickson ER, Lindor KD. Characteristics of patients with primary biliary cirrhosis (PBC) having a complete biochemical response to ursodiol. Gastroenterology. 1993;104:A923.
12. Combes B, Carithers RL, McDonald MF *et al*. Ursodeoxycholic acid therapy in patients with primary biliary cirrhosis. Hepatology. 1991;14:91A.
13. Podda M, Ghezzi C, Battezzati PM *et al*. Effect of different doses of ursodeoxycholic acid in chronic liver disease. Dig Dis Sci. 1989;34:59–65.

14. Stiehl A, Walker S, Stiehl L, Rudolph G, Hofmann WJ, Theilmann L. Effect of ursodeoxy-cholic acid on liver and bile duct disease in primary sclerosing cholangitis. A 3-year pilot study with a placebo-controlled study period. J Hepatol. 1994;20:57–64.
15. Lindor KD, Jorgensen RA, Anderson ML, Gores GJ, LaRusso NF. Ursodeoxycholic acid (UDCA) and methotrexate (MTX) for primary sclerosing cholangitis (PSC): a pilot study. Hepatology. 1994;20:148A.

17
Ursodeoxycholic acid in cholestatic liver diseases: clinical efficacy and putative mechanisms of action

R. POUPON, P. PODEVIN and R. E. POUPON

INTRODUCTION

Cholestasis can be defined as the clinical, biochemical and histological manifestations of defective bile acid transport from the liver to the intestine. Chronic cholestatic conditions of the liver form a homogeneous group of diseases with several points in common. Most result from the destruction of intrahepatic or extrahepatic bile ducts, or a developmental defect. Most chronic cholestatic conditions can progress towards cirrhosis (biliary cirrhosis) and hepatocellular insufficiency.

The rate of progression towards the terminal stage varies from patient to patient and depends on the nature of each disease and probably on the degree of bile duct destruction. For example, in PBC, follow-up studies of patients in controlled trials have shown that, within about 4 years, approximately 40% develop cirrhosis and 20% reach the terminal stage requiring transplantation[1]. Very similar results have been reported in sclerosing cholangitis[2-4]. Most children with bile duct atresia develop liver failure before the age of 3 years if they do not receive a transplant.

Terminal-stage chronic cholestatic conditions are an ideal indication for liver transplantation. This transforms the prognosis, giving a 5-year survival rate of about 70–80% if it is performed in good conditions.

RATIONALE FOR THE USE OF UDCA IN CHOLESTATIC DISORDERS

UDCA ($3\alpha,7\beta$-dihydroxy-5β-cholanic acid) is a natural bile acid in many mammals, but is only present in very small quantities in humans. UDCA is formed by 7β-epimerization of chenodeoxycholic acid, one of the two principal human bile acids, by certain intestinal organisms. Given its structural similarities

to chenodeoxycholic acid, it was postulated that it might also dissolve cholesterol gallstones, and this was confirmed in therapeutic trials. Two lessons were
learned from these trials: first, UDCA was capable of modifying the composition
of circulating bile acids in humans, becoming the predominant bile acid species;
and second, it was found to have no toxicity whatsoever, in contrast to chenodeoxycholic acid[5–7].

There are several lines of evidence that the defective bile acid elimination in
cholestatic conditions could be responsible for a major part of the clinical, biochemical and histopathological manifestations, as well as their progression
towards cirrhosis and hepatocellular failure. During the course of chronic
cholestatic conditions, bile acids accumulate in the liver, the systemic circulation
and peripheral tissue[8–11]. In the liver, concentrations close to 500–600 nmol/g
are sometimes observed. Since the pioneering work of Holsti[12], it has been
shown repeatedly that bile acids are hepatotoxic when administered to animals,
the isolated perfused liver or hepatocyte cultures. When given chronically to
certain animal species, they induce ductular lesions, fibrosis and even cirrhosis[13]. In humans, the administration of chenodeoxycholic and deoxycholic acids
can increase transaminase activity and lead to histological changes in the
liver[14,15]. The toxic effects of bile acids include a series of phenomena observed
during cholestasis and *in vitro*: increased membrane fluidity, increased membrane permeability (especially to calcium), impaired oxidative phosphorylation,
decreased mono-oxygenase activities, inhibition of γ-glutamyl transpeptidase
and glutathione transferase activities, changes in cytoskeleton organization,
induction of free-radical injury, changes in DNA superstructure and, finally, cell
apoptosis and necrosis. These deleterious effects apparently are influenced by
three main factors: (a) the chemical structure and the degree of hydrophobicity
of the bile acid; (b) the nature of the cells or tissue exposed to bile acids; and
(c) the concentration–time product in or around the cells.

Contrary to endogenous human bile acids and, particularly, chenodeoxycholic
acid, UDCA is strongly hydrophilic and is not toxic *in vitro* or in humans. In
particular, UDCA has no toxicity up to concentrations of 500 μmol/L in several
in-vitro models. In humans, UDCA is at least partly transformed into lithocholic
acid. However, humans rapidly detoxify and excrete lithocholate, which therefore does not accumulate in the enterohepatic circulation[16].

Although we do not know precisely how bile acid accumulation damages the
liver, it is now possible to sketch a simplified mechanism of action of UDCA in
cholestasis. UDCA inhibits the intestinal absorption and increases the canalicular excretion of cholic and chenodeoxycholic acids. Inhibition of bile acid
intestinal absorption is well documented. During UDCA therapy, the fractional
turn-over rate and ileal excretion of cholic and chenodeoxycholic acids increase.
However, several lines of evidence suggest that decreased intestinal absorption
is not the only explanation for the hepatoprotective effect of UDCA in cholestasis. For example, cholestyramine, which also reduces bile acid concentrations,
does not have frank beneficial effects in chronic cholestatic conditions. Indeed,
several lines of evidence suggest that UDCA protects the liver through an
increase in the intrinsic ability to secrete bile acids and other organic anions into
bile. The mechanisms of this peculiar property is discussed elsewere in detail.
Other possible mechanisms involve immune modulation – UDCA reduces both

cholestasis and abnormal expression of HLA Class I molecules on hepatocytes[17,18], and also possibly on biliary cells – and stabilization of hepatocellular membranes[19,20].

TREATMENT OF ADULT CHOLESTATIC DISORDERS

Primary biliary cirrhosis

Immunosuppressive treatments have been used in controlled trials for the treatment of PBC. Colchicine has been used for its antifibrotic and anti-inflammatory properties. Most of these drugs, especially cyclosporin, had a certain effect on laboratory measures but not on the prognosis of the disease.

In 1987, we postulated that long-term treatment with UDCA might displace endogenous bile acids and thus, reverse their suspected cytotoxicity. In a pilot study of patients with PBC, UDCA indeed led to major sustained improvements in liver function tests[21]. To determine whether UDCA would slow the progression of PBC towards the terminal phase, we conducted a 2-year multicentre double-blind, controlled trial in which patients with PBC were randomized to receive either UDCA or a placebo[22]. Patients were admitted to the trial regardless of the duration of the symptoms and histological severity. The end-point chosen to define failure of UDCA treatment was one of the following criteria: hyperbilirubinaemia, clinical complication (variceal bleeding, ascites, encephalopathy) or a major adverse effect. Following randomization, 73 patients with PBC received UDCA ($13–15$ mgkg^{-1}d^{-1}) and 73 the placebo. At entry, the two groups were well matched for age, sex, time since initial diagnosis and histological severity: in the UDCA group, 50% of the patients had Stage I–II disease, compared with 56% in the placebo group. At the end of the trial, the risk of failure was significantly (about 3-fold) higher in the placebo group than in the UDCA group. One patient in each group withdrew because of adverse effects. After 2 years of treatment, the proportion of treated patients with clinically overt disease had fallen significantly; in particular, there was a clear improvement in terms of the severity of pruritus. Patients receiving UDCA showed significant improvements in serum bilirubin level, alkaline phosphatase, transaminases, γ-glutamyl transpeptidase activities, cholesterol and immunoglobulin M levels, the anti-mitochondrial antibody titer and the Mayo risk score. There was a significant improvement in the mean histological score and in all the histological features, except fibrosis, only in the group given UDCA.

Because of the patient selection and the short duration of follow-up, there were few liver transplantations, preventing any comparison between the two groups of treatment on the basis of this criterion[22]. Given the benefit of UDCA, patients completing the study received UDCA in an open fashion and were monitored for a further 2 years. At 4 years, there had been 4 liver transplantations in the original UDCA group, compared with 13 in the original placebo group. The incidence of liver transplantation was significantly lower in the patients who received UDCA for 4 years than in those initially receiving the placebo ($p = 0.003$, relative risk = 0.21 (CI = 0.09–0.76)). Thus, long-term UDCA therapy slows the progression of the disease[23].

During the study period, other trials of UDCA in PBC were set up[24–28]. The data so far available consistently show an improvement in biochemical parameters. By contrast, improvements in clinical and histological parameters are inconsistently found; however, it must be underlined that these trials lack the power required to conclude that UDCA has no effect on these parameters. The recent results of two large North American trials[29,30] indicate that UDCA delayed the progression of the disease but without reducing the need for liver transplantation. The apparent discrepancies with our results could be related to the duration of treatment and/or the selection of patients. Analysis of the combined data of these two trials and ours (550 patients) confirms that four-year UDCA treatment decreases the risk of liver transplantation and death[31].

Primary sclerosing cholangitis

Since sclerosing cholangitis and PBC share certain features, we studied the clinical and biochemical effects of UDCA administration in patients with sclerosing cholangitis[32]. In an uncontrolled study (15 patients given 8–16 mgkg^{-1}d^{-1} UDCA), the proportion of patients suffering from fatigue or pruritus after 6 months of treatment fell from 60% to 20% and from 33% to 20%, respectively. Serum activities of alkaline phosphatases, γ-glutamyl transpeptidase and transaminases also fell significantly. No exacerbation of associated disorders or side-effects of UDCA were observed. The efficacy of UDCA was suggested by:

1. The clear improvement in patients in whom the cholestasis had been stable for at least 6 months,
2. The absence of similar spontaneous improvements during the natural history of the disease, and
3. Aggravation of liver test results following the discontinuation of UDCA in three patients.

Two other pilot studies have confirmed these results. One[33], in which 12 patients were treated for a mean period of 30 months with 10 mgkg^{-1}d^{-1} UDCA, confirmed the improvement of biochemical test results after six months of treatment, and the further improvement with long-term treatment. The other[34], in which 22 patients received UDCA for one year and were then randomized to receive either UDCA or a placebo for a further year, was interrupted for ethical reasons, i.e. the aggravation of disease in patients receiving the placebo. Similar results were reported by Beuers *et al.*[18]: in a placebo-controlled trial, UDCA was found to reduce disease activity in patients with sclerosing cholangitis. After one year of treatment, the patients in the UDCA group showed improvements relative to the placebo group with respect to serum levels of bilirubin, alkaline phosphatase, γ-glutamyl transpeptidase and transaminases. Histological features, evaluated with a multiparametric score, also improved.

Although the effectiveness of UDCA in sclerosing cholangitis has been demonstrated, it is less valuable in this condition than in PBC. Indeed, patients with sclerosing cholangitis frequently develop a cholangiocarcinoma and liver transplantation is more widely indicated than in PBC; thus, UDCA therapy is aimed mainly at obtaining an improvement in the quality of life and in the patient's condition, with a view to transplantation.

Intrahepatic cholestasis of pregnancy

Intrahepatic cholestasis of pregnancy is a condition of unknown origin, characterized by pruritus and abnormal liver test results, with a predominantly cholestatic pattern. It appears during the second half of pregnancy in previously healthy women. After delivery, the pruritus resolves rapidly and biochemical parameters return to normal. Besides the discomfort for the mothers, this disease causes an increased rate of fetal distress, premature delivery and perinatal mortality; there is no effective treatment.

In an open study, UDCA administration to eight patients with intrahepatic cholestasis of pregnancy led to an improvement in pruritus and laboratory test results. UDCA was well tolerated and had no apparent toxicity for either the mother or the child[35]. Unfortunately, data concerning bile acid composition before and during UDCA therapy were lacking.

In a case of triple pregnancy complicated by early cholestasis, UDCA administration normalized maternal liver function[36]. The marked improvement in clinical and biochemical parameters, including serum bile acid levels, suggests a role of endogenous bile acids in the onset of this form of cholestasis.

Other settings

Liver graft rejection

Acute and chronic liver graft rejection is a frequent complication of liver transplantation, affecting 50–75% of patients and justifying aggressive treatment. UDCA could be effective in this setting for the following reasons:

1. There is a striking similarity between the characteristic lesions of PBC and those of liver rejection,
2. In both cases, there is abnormal expression of Class I and II HLA molecules in the liver, and
3. Both conditions are associated with cholestasis and the destruction of interlobular bile ducts.

In PBC, UDCA reduces HLA Class I expression in the liver[17], prevents duct destruction and improves the cholestasis.

The results of a pilot study[37] are in favour of such an action. During the first month after liver transplantation, 2 episodes of rejection were observed in 18 consecutive patients who received UDCA, compared with 6 out of 8 previous patients who had received the usual immunosuppressive treatments. However, these results were not confirmed subsequently[38]. During the 6 months after liver transplantation, 12 rejection episodes were observed among 8 of 15 patients treated with UDCA, while 10 episodes occurred in 7 of 14 untreated patients. Unfortunately, the interpretation of these results is limited by the absence of randomization and the lack of data concerning the bioavailability of UDCA during the postoperative period.

Chronic graft-versus-host disease of the liver

The natural history of GVHD of the liver suggests that biliary cirrhosis may be the end stage. On the basis of biochemical, clinical and histological similarities between GVHD and PBC, the efficacy of UDCA was tested in the therapy of GVHD of the liver[39]. UDCA (10–15 mgkg^{-1}d^{-1}) was given for 6 weeks to 12 patients who had failed to respond to immunosuppressive therapy. Biochemical parameters were improved by UDCA and returned to pretreatment values after discontinuation of the treatment. This preliminary study required confirmation in longer-term controlled trials.

Cyclosporin-induced cholestasis

Cholestasis induced by cyclosporin A following liver transplantation may be improved by the administration of UDCA[40]. The study concerned 13 heart-transplant recipients, 5 of whom developed cholestasis during immunosuppressive therapy, including cyclosporin A. All 5 patients received UDCA; although no change in blood cyclosporin levels was observed, alkaline phosphatase, γ-glutamyl transpeptidase and transaminase activities, as well as bilirubinaemia, were markedly reduce. When UDCA was discontinued, all five patients redeveloped cholestasis, which again resolved when on UDCA.

Parenteral-nutrition-associated cholestasis

Cholestasis can occur during long-term parenteral nutrition, and no treatment is known to be effective. A case report and, very recently, a cross-over study, suggest that UDCA can prevent or improve abnormalities in liver tests in this setting[11,12].

Benign recurrent intrahepatic cholestasis

Benign recurrent intrahepatic cholestasis is characterized by the abrupt onset of severe cholestasis, which spontaneously subsides after several weeks in otherwise healthy subjects. These acute attacks have been attributed to unknown factors impairing bile acid transport at the canalicular level in genetically susceptible subjects. All treatments so far evaluated have proven unsatisfactory. Recently, a contracted bile acid pool size was reported in these patients[43] and thus the use of UDCA was suggested. On the basis of a detailed clinical report, it appears that UDCA is unable to prevent acute cholestatic episodes[44]. In contrast, in a case report, UDCA was found to have a beneficial effect over 4 years[45]. However, because the course of this disease is highly variable, it is difficult to prove or disprove the efficacy of UDCA.

TREATMENT OF CHILDHOOD CHOLESTATIC DISEASES

Cystic fibrosis

With the improved efficacy of treatments for pulmonary conditions, the survival of patients with cystic fibrosis has increased considerably. In contrast, hepatobiliary complications are more and more frequent: about 25% of adult patients have biliary abnormalities which, in 5–10% of the cases, progress to cirrhosis.

In young patients with cystic fibrosis and severe cholestasis, UDCA not only improved conventional liver tests, but also improved nutritional parameters[46,47].

As in other cholestatic diseases, it seems likely that the beneficial effect of UDCA on cholestasis involves similar mechanisms, including an improvement in hepatic excretory function[47,48] and, as a possible consequence, an improvement in biliary drainage. In contrast, why UDCA should act on nutritional status is less clear. An improvement in intestinal fat absorption can be ruled out because of the lack of change in faecal fat excretion[49], and the fact that UDCA inhibits intestinal cholesterol absorption. The most reasonable hypothesis is that nutritional status improves following improvement in liver function.

Other childhood cholestatic diseases

Controlled studies are currently underway to evaluate the effects of UDCA in intrahepatic bile duct paucity syndromes, including Alagille syndrome and Byler disease[50]. Preliminary results show that UDCA has a spectacular effect on pruritus, laboratory test results, jaundice and nutritional status. Similar effects have been reported in patients with extrahepatic bile duct atresia[51,52], in whom treatment with UDCA enabled Kasai's operation to be performed in excellent conditions.

Inborn errors of bile acid metabolism

Childhood cholestatic diseases, characterized by errors of bile acid synthesis (3β-hydroxysteroid dehydrogenase and Δ^4-3-oxosteroid-5-α-reductase deficits; Zellweger syndrome) manifest clinically as neonatal cholestasis, which can progress towards cirrhosis and death, and biologically as a predominance of atypical bile acids[53]. Cholestasis could result from either the inability of the liver to synthesize primary bile acids (essential for bile secretion) or from the toxicity of the atypical bile acids. Treatment with UDCA together with cholate and/or chenodeoxycholate could be effective[54].

CONCLUSION

Until the 1980s, the role of bile acids in the initiation of liver injury in humans was only suspected on the basis of the toxicity of whole bile and bile salts and studies showing elevations in serum and tissue levels of bile salts in liver diseases. The beneficial effects of UDCA in PBC have provided the first firm evidence that, in some way, bile acids may be related to liver injury in humans.

These observations raise a series of questions and challenges in clinical, cellular and molecular research. For example, is UDCA capable of modifying the progression and prognosis of other cholestatic conditions of children and adults and, more generally, liver diseases in which the enterohepatic bile acid circulation is disturbed? Is it possible and warranted to design UDCA analogues with stronger activities and more specific targets? And how might UDCA and these analogues modulate fundamental cell or organelle functions and cell-to-cell relationships in the normal and cholestatic liver?

References

1. Christensen E, Crowe J, Doniach D *et al*. Clinical pattern and course of disease in primary biliary cirrhosis based on an analysis of 236 patients. Gastroenterology. 1980;78:236–46.

2. Dickson ER, Murtaugh PA, Wiesner RH *et al.* (1992). Primary sclerosing cholangitis: refinement and validation of survival models. Gastroenterology. 1992;103:1893–901.

3. LaRusso NF, Weisner RH, Ludwig J *et al.* Prospective trial of penicillamine in primary sclerosing cholangitis. Gastroenterology. 1988;95:1036–42.

4. Weisner RH, Grambsch PM, Dickson ER *et al.* Primary sclerosing cholangitis: natural history, prognostic factors and survival analysis. Hepatology. 1989;10:430–6.

5. Bachrach WH, Hofmann AF. Ursodeoxycholic acid in the treatment of cholesterol cholelithiasis. Part I. Dig Dis Sci. 1982;24:737–61.

6. Bachrach WH, Hofmann AF. Ursodeoxycholic acid in the treatment of cholesterol cholelithiasis. Part II. Dig Dis Sci. 1982;24:833–56.

7. Poupon RE, Poupon R. Ursodeoxycholic acid for treatment of cholestatic diseases. In: Boyer JL, Ockner RK, eds. Progress in liver diseases. Eastbourne, UK; WB Saunders Company; 1992:219–38.

8. Greim H, Czygan P, Schaffner F, Popper H. Determination of bile acids in needle biopsies of human liver. Biochem Med. 1973;8:280–6.

9. Akashi Y, Miyazaki H, Yanagisawa J, Nakayama F. Bile acid metabolism in cirrhotic liver tissue-altered synthesis and impaired hepatic secretion. Clin Chim Acta. 1987;168:199–206.

10. Hendenborg G, Norlander A, Norman A. Bile acid conjugates presents in tissues during extrahepatic cholestasis. Scand J Clin Lab Invest. 1986;46:539–44.

11. Dupont J, Garcia PA, Hennig B *et al.* Bile acids in extrahepatic tissues. In: Setchell KDR, Kritchevsky D, Nair PP, eds. The bile acids: Chemistry, physiology, and metabolism New York and London: Plenum Press; 1987:341–69.

12. Holsti P. Experimental cirrhosis of the liver in rabbits induced by gastric instillation of dessicated whole bile. Acta Path Microbiol Scand. 1956;112:1–67.

13. Palmer RH. Bile acids, liver injury, and liver disease. Arch Intern Med. 1972;130:606–17.

14. LaRusso NF, Szczepanik PA, Hofmann AF. Effect of deoxycholic acid ingestion on bile acid metabolism and biliary lipid secretion in normal subjects. Gastroenterology. 1977;72:132–40.

15. Schoenfield LJ, Lachin JM. Chenodiol (chenodeoxycholic acid) for dissolution of gallstones: the National Cooperative Gallstone Study: a controlled trial of efficacy and safety. Ann Intern Med. 1981;95:257–82.

16. Cowen AC, Korman MG, Hofmann AF, Cass OW, Coffin SB (1975). Metabolism of litho cholate in healthy man. Gastroenterology. 1975;69:62–76.

17. Calmus Y, Gane P, Rouger P, Poupon R. Hepatic expression of class I and class II major histocompatibility complex molecules in primary biliary cirrhosis: effect of ursodeoxycholic acid. Hepatology. 1990;11:12–15.

18. Beuers U, Spengler U, Kruis W *et al.* Ursodeoxycholic acid for treatment of primary sclerosing cholangitis: a placebo-controlled trial. Hepatology. 1992;16:707–14.

19. Güldütuna S, Immer G, Imohof BS, You T, Leuschner U. Molecular aspects of membrane stabilization by ursodeoxycholate. Gastroenterology. 1993;104:1736–44.

20. Heuman DM. Hepatoprotective properties of ursodeoxycholic acid. Gastroenterology. 1993;104:1865–70.

21. Poupon R, Chrétien Y, Poupon RE *et al.* Is ursodeoxycholic acid an effective treatment for primary biliary cirrhosis? Lancet. 1987;1:834–6.

22. Poupon RE, Balkau B, Eschwège E, Poupon R and the UDCA-PBC Study Group. A multicenter, controlled trial of ursodiol for the treatment of primary biliary cirrhosis. N Engl J Med. 1991;324:1548–54.

23. Poupon RE, Poupon R, Balkau B and the UDCA-PBC Study Group. Ursodiol for the long-term treatment of primary biliary cirrhosis. N Engl J Med. 1994;330:1342–7.

24. Leuschner U, Fischer H, Kurtz W *et al.* Ursodeoxycholic acid in primary biliary cirrhosis – Results of a controlled double-blind trial. Gastroenterology. 1989;97:1268–74.

25. Oka H, Toda G, Ikeda Y *et al.* A multicenter double-blind controlled trial of ursodeoxycholic acid for primary biliary cirrhosis. Gastroenterol Jpn. 1990;25:774–80.

26. Combes B, Carithers RL, MacDonald MF *et al.* Ursodeoxycholic acid in patients with primary biliary cirrhosis. Hepatology. 1991;14:91.

27. Battezzati P, Podda M, Bianchi F *et al.* Ursodeoxycholic acid for symptomatic primary biliary cirrhosis – Preliminary analysis of a double-blind multicenter trial. J Hepatol. 1993;17:332–8.

28. Turner IB, Myszor M, Mitchison HC *et al.* A two year controlled trial examining the effectiveness of ursodeoxycholic acid in primary biliary cirrhosis. J Gastroenterol Hepatol. 1994;9:162–8.

29. Heathcote EJ, Cauch-Dubek K, Walker V *et al.* The Canadian multicenter double-blind randomized controlled trial of ursodeoxycholic acid in primary biliary cirrhosis. Hepatology. 1994;19:1149–56.
30. Lindor KD, Dickson ER, Baldus WP *et al.* Ursodeoxycholic acid in the treatment of primary biliary cirrhosis. Gastroenterology. 1994;106:1284–90.
31. Heathcote EJ, Lindor KD, Poupon R *et al.* Combined analysis of French, American and Canadian randomized trials of ursodeoxycholic acid therapy in primary biliary cirrhosis. Gastroenterology. 1995;108:1086(abstr.).
32. Chazouillères O, Poupon R, Capron JP *et al.* Ursodeoxycholic acid for primary sclerosing cholangitis. J Hepatol. 1990;11:120–3.
33. O'Brien CB, Senior JR, Arora-Mirchandani R, Batta AK, Salen G. Ursodeoxycholic acid for the treatment of primary sclerosing cholangitis: a 30-month pilot study. Hepatology. 1991;14:838–47.
34. Stiehl A, Walker S, Stiehl L *et al.* Effect of ursodeoxycholic acid on liver and bile duct disease in primary sclerosing cholangitis. A 3-year pilot study with a placebo-controlled study period. J Hepatol. 1994;20:57–64.
35. Palma J, Reyes JH, Ribalta J *et al.* Effects of ursodeoxycholic acid in patients with intrahepatic cholestasis of pregnancy. Hepatology. 1992;15:1043–7.
36. Marpeau L, Chazouillères O, Rhimi Z *et al.* Pregnancy-associated idiopathic intrahepatic cholestasis. Hypotheses of physiopathology: a therapeutic case report. Fetal Diagn Ther. 1991;6:120–5.
37. Svanvik J, Frimman S, Persson H, Schertén T, Karlberg I. Does adjuvant ursodeoxycholic acid prevent acute rejection in liver transplant recipients? In: Paumgartner G, Stiehl A, Gerok W, eds. Bile acids as therapeutic agents. Lancaster, UK: Kluwer Academic Publishers; 1990;357–60.
38. Sama C, Mazzioti A, Grigioni W, *et al.* Ursodeoxycholic acid administration does not prevent rejection after OLT. J Hepatol. 1991;13:68(abstr.)
39. Fried RH, Murakami CS, Fisher LD, *et al.* Ursodeoxycholic acid treatment of refractory chronic graft-versus-host disease of the liver. Ann Intern Med. 1992;116:624–9.
40. Kallinowski B, Theilmann L, Zimmermann R, *et al.* Effective treatment of cyclosporine-induced cholestasis in heart-transplanted patients treated with ursodeoxycholic acid. Transplantation. 1991;51:1128–9.
41. Lindor KD, Burnes J. Ursodeoxycholic acid for the treatment of home parenteral nutrition associated cholestasis – A case report. Gastroenterology. 1991;101:250–3.
42. Beau P, Labat-Labourdette J, Ingrand P, Beauchant M. Is ursodeoxycholic acid an effective therapy for total parenteral nutrition-related liver disease? J Hepatol. 1994;20:240–4.
43. Bijleveld C, Vonk R, Kuipers F *et al.* Benign recurrent intrahepatic cholestasis: altered bile acid metabolism. Gastroenterology. 1989;97:427–32.
44. Crosignani A, Podda M, Bertoloni E *et al.* Failure of ursodeoxycholic acid to prevent a cholestatic episode in a patient with benign recurrent intrahepatic cholestasis: a study of bile acid metabolism. Hepatology. 1991;13:1076–83.
45. Maggiore G, De Giacomo C. Efficacy of ursodeoxycholic acid in preventing cholestatic episodes in a patient with benign recurrent intrahepatic cholestasis. Hepatology. 1992;16:504 (Letter).
46. Colombo C, Setchell K, Podda M *et al.* Effects of ursodeoxycholic acid therapy for liver disease associated with cystic fibrosis. J Pediatr. 1990;117:482–9.
47. Cotting J, Dufour J, Lentze M, Paumgartner G, Reichen J. Ursodeoxycholate in the treatment of cholestatis in cystic fibrosis. A two-year experience and review of the literature. In: Lentze M, Reichen J, eds. Paediatric cholestasis. Novel approaches to treatment. Lancaster, UK: Kluwer Academic Publishers; 1992:345–53.
48. Colombo C, Crosignani A, Assaisso M *et al.* Ursodeoxycholic acid therapy in cystic fibrosis associated liver disease – A dose–response study. Hepatology. 1992;16:924–30.
49. Bittner P, Posselt HG, Sailer T *et al.* The effect of ursodeoxycholic acid in cystic fibrosis and hepatopathy: results of a placebo-controlled study. In: Paumgartner G, Stiehl A, Gerok W, eds. Bile acids as therapeutic agents. Lancaster, UK: Kluwer Academic Publishers; 1990:345–56.
50. Balistreri WF, A-Kader HH, Ryckman FC *et al.* Biochemical and clinical response to ursodeoxycholic acid administration in paediatric patients with chronic cholestasis. In: Paumgartner G, Stiehl A, Gerok W, eds. Bile acids as therapeutic agents. Lancaster, UK: Kluwer Academic Publishers; 1990:323–33.

51. Nittono H, Tokita A, Hayashi M *et al.* Ursodeoxycholic acid in biliary atresia. Lancet. 1988;1:528(Letter)
52. Ullrich D, Rating D, Schröter W, Hanefeld F, Bircher J. Treatment with ursodeoxycholic acid renders children with biliary atresia suitable for liver transplantation. Lancet. 1987;2:1324(Letter).
53. Setchell KDR, Bragetti P, Zimmer-Nechemias L *et al.* Oral bile acid treatment and the patient with Zellweger syndrome. Hepatology. 1992;15:198–207.
54. Daugherty CC, Setchell KDR, Heubi JE, Balistreri WF. Resolution of liver biopsy alterations in three siblings with bile acid treatment of an inborn error of bile acid metabolism (Δ4-3-oxosteroid 5β-reductase deficiency). Hepatology. 1993;18:1096–101.

Index

Falk Symposium Series

43. Reutter W, Popper H, Arias IM, Heinrich PC, Keppler D, Landmann L, eds.: *Modulation of Liver Cell Expression*. Falk Symposium No. 43. 1987   ISBN: 0-85200-677-2*

44. Boyer JL, Bianchi L, eds.: *Liver Cirrhosis*. Falk Symposium No. 44. 1987
   ISBN: 0-85200-993-3*

45. Paumgartner G, Stiehl A, Gerok W, eds.: *Bile Acids and the Liver*. Falk Symposium No. 45. 1987   ISBN: 0-85200-675-6*

46. Goebell H, Peskar BM, Malchow H, eds.: *Inflammatory Bowel Diseases – Basic Research & Clinical Implications*. Falk Symposium No. 46. 1988   ISBN: 0-7462-0067-6*

47. Bianchi L, Holt P, James OFW, Butler RN, eds.: *Aging in Liver and Gastrointestinal Tract*. Falk Symposium No. 47. 1988   ISBN: 0-7462-0066-8*

48. Heilmann C, ed.: *Calcium-Dependent Processes in the Liver*. Falk Symposium No. 48. 1988   ISBN: 0-7462-0075-7*

50. Singer MV, Goebell H, eds.: *Nerves and the Gastrointestinal Tract*. Falk Symposium No. 50. 1989   ISBN: 0-7462-0114-1

51. Bannasch P, Keppler D, Weber G, eds.: *Liver Cell Carcinoma*. Falk Symposium No. 51. 1989   ISBN: 0-7462-0111-7

52. Paumgartner G, Stiehl A, Gerok W, eds.: *Trends in Bile Acid Research*. Falk Symposium No. 52. 1989   ISBN: 0-7462-0112-5

53. Paumgartner G, Stiehl A, Barbara L, Roda E, eds.: *Strategies for the Treatment of Hepatobiliary Diseases*. Falk Symposium No. 53. 1990   ISBN: 0-7923-8903-4

54. Bianchi L, Gerok W, Maier K-P, Deinhardt F, eds.: *Infectious Diseases of the Liver*. Falk Symposium No. 54. 1990   ISBN: 0-7923-8902-6

55. Falk Symposium No. 55 not published

55B. Hadziselimovic F, Herzog B, Bürgin-Wolff A, eds.: *Inflammatory Bowel Disease and Coeliac Disease in Children*. International Falk Symposium. 1990 ISBN 0-7462-0125-7

56. Williams CN, eds.: *Trends in Inflammatory Bowel Disease Therapy*. Falk Symposium No. 56. 1990   ISBN: 0-7923-8952-2

57. Bock KW, Gerok W, Matern S, Schmid R, eds.: *Hepatic Metabolism and Disposition of Endo- and Xenobiotics*. Falk Symposium No. 57. 1991   ISBN: 0-7923-8953-0

58. Paumgartner G, Stiehl A, Gerok W, eds.: *Bile Acids as Therapeutic Agents: From Basic Science to Clinical Practice*. Falk Symposium No. 58. 1991   ISBN: 0-7923-8954-9

59. Halter F, Garner A, Tytgat GNJ, eds.: *Mechanisms of Peptic Ulcer Healing*. Falk Symposium No. 59. 1991   ISBN: 0-7923-8955-7

60. Goebell H, Ewe K, Malchow H, Koelbel Ch, eds.: *Inflammatory Bowel Diseases – Progress in Basic Research and Clinical Implications*. Falk Symposium No. 60. 1991
   ISBN: 0-7923-8956-5

61. Falk Symposium No. 61 not published

62. Dowling RH, Folsch UR, Löser Ch, eds.: *Polyamines in the Gastrointestinal Tract*. Falk Symposium No. 62. 1992   ISBN: 0-7923-8976-X

63. Lentze MJ, Reichen J, eds.: *Paediatric Cholestasis: Novel Approaches to Treatment*. Falk Symposium No. 63. 1992   ISBN: 0-7923-8977-8

64. Demling L, Frühmorgen P, eds.: *Non-Neoplastic Diseases of the Anorectum*. Falk Symposium No. 64. 1992   ISBN: 0-7923-8979-4

64B. Gressner AM, Ramadori G, eds.: *Molecular and Cell Biology of Liver Fibrogenesis*. International Falk Symposium. 1992   ISBN: 0-7923-8980-8

*These titles were published under the MTP Press imprint.

Falk Symposium Series

65. Hadziselimovic F, Herzog B, eds.: *Inflammatory Bowel Diseases and Morbus Hirschprung.* Falk Symposium No. 65. 1992   ISBN: 0-7923-8995-6

66. Martin F, McLeod RS, Sutherland LR, Williams CN, eds.: *Trends in Inflammatory Bowel Disease Therapy.* Falk Symposium No. 66. 1993   ISBN: 0-7923-8827-5

67. Schölmerich J, Kruis W, Goebell H, Hohenberger W, Gross V, eds.: *Inflammatory Bowel Diseases – Pathophysiology as Basis of Treatment.* Falk Symposium No. 67. 1993
ISBN: 0-7923-8996-4

68. Paumgartner G, Stiehl A, Gerok W, eds.: *Bile Acids and The Hepatobiliary System: From Basic Science to Clinical Practice.* Falk Symposium No. 68. 1993
ISBN: 0-7923-8829-1

69. Schmid R, Bianchi L, Gerok W, Maier K-P, eds.: *Extrahepatic Manifestations in Liver Diseases.* Falk Symposium No. 69. 1993   ISBN: 0-7923-8821-6

70. Meyer zum Büschenfelde K-H, Hoofnagle J, Manns M, eds.: *Immunology and Liver.* Falk Symposium No. 70. 1993   ISBN: 0-7923-8830-5

71. Surrenti C, Casini A, Milani S, Pinzani M , eds.: *Fat-Storing Cells and Liver Fibrosis.* Falk Symposium No. 71. 1994   ISBN: 0-7923-8842-9

72. Rachmilewitz D, ed.: *Inflammatory Bowel Diseases – 1994.* Falk Symposium No. 72. 1994   ISBN: 0-7923-8845-3

73. Binder HJ, Cummings J, Soergel KH, eds.: *Short Chain Fatty Acids.* Falk Symposium No. 73. 1994   ISBN: 0-7923-8849-6

74. Keppler D, Jungermann K, eds.: *Transport in the Liver.* Falk Symposium No. 74. 1994
ISBN: 0-7923-8858-5

74B. Stange EF, ed.: *Chronic Inflammatory Bowel Disease.* Falk Symposium. 1995
ISBN: 0-7923-8876-3

75. van Berge Henegouwen GP, van Hoek B, De Groote J, Matern S, Stockbrügger RW, eds.: *Cholestatic Liver Diseases: New Strategies for Prevention and Treatment of Hepatobiliary and Cholestatic Liver Diseases.* Falk Symposium 75. 1994.
ISBN: 0-7923-8867-4

76. Monteiro E, Tavarela Veloso F, eds.: *Inflammatory Bowel Diseases: New Insights into Mechanisms of Inflammation and Challenges in Diagnosis and Treatment.* Falk Symposium 76. 1995.   ISBN 0-7923-8884-4

77. Singer MV, Ziegler R, Rohr G, eds.: *Gastrointestinal Tract and Endocrine System.* Falk Symposium 77. 1995.   ISBN 0-7923-8877-1

78. Decker K, Gerok W, Andus T, Gross V, eds.: *Cytokines and the Liver.* Falk Symposium 78. 1995.   ISBN 0-7923-8878-X

79. Holstege A, Schölmerich J, Hahn EG, eds.: *Portal Hypertension.* Falk Symposium 79. 1995.   ISBN 0-7923-8879-8

80. Hofmann AF, Paumgartner G, Stiehl A, eds.: *Bile Acids in Gastroenterology: Basic and Clinical Aspects.* Falk Symposium 80. 1995   ISBN 0-7923-8880-1

81. Riecken EO, Stallmach A, Zeitz M, Heise W, eds.: *Malignancy and Chronic Inflammation in the Gastrointestinal Tract – New Concepts.* Falk Symposium 81. 1995
ISBN 0-7923-8889-5

82. Fleig WE, ed.: *Inflammatory Bowel Diseases: New Developments and Standards.* Falk Symposium 82. 1995   ISBN 0-7923-8890-6

82B. Paumgartner G, Beuers U, eds.: *Bile Acids in Liver Diseases.* International Falk Workshop. 1995   ISBN 0-7923-8891-7

83. Dobrilla G, Felder M, de Pretis G, eds.: *Advances in Hepatobiliary and Pancreatic Diseases: Special Clinical Topics.* Falk Symposium 83. 1995.   ISBN 0-7923-8892-5

Falk Symposium Series

84. Fromm H, Leuschner U, eds.: *Bile Acids – Cholestasis – Gallstones: Advances in Basic and Clinical Bile Acid Research.* Falk Symposium 84. 1995   ISBN 0-7923-8893-3
85. Tytgat GNJ, Bartelsman JFWM, van Deventer SJH, eds.: *Inflammatory Bowel Diseases.* Falk Symposium 85. 1995   ISBN 0-7923-8894-1